DIGESTIVE DISEASES - RESEARCH AND CLINICAL DEVELOPMENTS

INTUSSUSCEPTION AND BOWEL OBSTRUCTION

SYMPTOMS, DIAGNOSIS AND TREATMENT OPTIONS

DIGESTIVE DISEASES - RESEARCH AND CLINICAL DEVELOPMENTS

Additional books in this series can be found on Nova's website under the Series tab.

Additional e-books in this series can be found on Nova's website under the e-book tab.

DIGESTIVE DISEASES - RESEARCH AND CLINICAL DEVELOPMENTS

INTUSSUSCEPTION AND BOWEL OBSTRUCTION

SYMPTOMS, DIAGNOSIS AND TREATMENT OPTIONS

ROSIE MILLER
EDITOR

New York

Library of Congress Cataloging-in-Publication Data

ISBN: 978-1-63482-703-4

Library of Congress Control Number: 2015937676

Published by Nova Science Publishers, Inc. † New York

Contents

Preface		**vii**
Chapter 1	Intussusception: Symptoms *T. Dionysis and P. Petropoulos*	**1**
Chapter 2	Rectal Intussusception and Its Clinical Spectrum *Sanjay Harrison and Harrison Benziger*	**9**
Chapter 3	Japanese Guidelines for Intussusceptions and Current Management *Yasuo Ito*	**31**
Chapter 4	Prenatal Intussusception: What Consequences? *Taieb Chouikh, Chaima Mrad, Awatef Charieg, Sofiene Ghorbel and Sonia Benkhalifa*	**77**
Chapter 5	Laparoscopic Treatment of Intussusception *Philip E. George and Edward Chin*	**87**
Chapter 6	Afferent Loop Obstruction *K. Blouhos, K. A. Boulas, K. Tsalis and A. Hatzigeorgiadis*	**97**
Chapter 7	Decreasing Post-Surgical Adhesions That Cause Recurrent Small Bowel Obstructions with a Conservative Manual Physical Therapy *Amanda D. Rice and C. Richard King*	**113**

Chapter 8 Alternative Treatment of Non-Malignant Bowel Obstruction in Patients with Gynecological Cancer **125**
C. Richard King, III and Amanda D. Rice

Index **141**

Preface

Intussusception is the most frequent cause of bowel obstruction in infants and toddlers. In this book, the symptoms and clinical findings of intussuception are discussed. The clinical guidelines for the management of intussuceptions in children are discussed as well. Other chapters examine the diagnosis, etiology, pathophysiology and treatment modalities for both small bowel obstruction and intussusception of the small bowel, focusing on minimally invasive surgical options; the etiology of afferent loop obstruction; the treatment options for adhesive small bowel obstruction (SBO), a common complication typically caused by adhesions that form after abdominal surgery; a literature review of traditional medical treatment options and a discussion on the authors' experiences in treating gynecological cancer patients with non-malignant bowel obstruction using manual physical therapy.

Chapter 1 – Intussusception is the most frequent cause of bowel obstruction in infants and toddlers. It is an acquired invagination of the proximal bowel (intussusceptum) into the distal bowel (intussuscipiens). The classic presentation is an infant or a young child with intermittent, crampy abdominal pain associated with 'currant jelly' stools and a palpable mass on physical examination, although this triad is seen in less than a fourth of children. Vomiting is seen in 80 per cent; this maybe an early reflex feature or bilious if complete obstruction has occurred. Infants present more often with vomiting than older children do (up to 45%). Bilious vomiting tends to be found in delayed cases of intussusception with SBO. Occasionally, infants will present to the admitting pediatrician with severe lethargy and features suggestive of meningitis. The absence of pain, however, does not rule out intussusceptions but may delay the diagnosis. It is important to know that about 15% of infants and children present without any obvious pain. These children are often pale and listless and appear quite ill. In this chapter, the authors develop the symptoms and clinical findings of the intussusception.

Chapter 2 – Introduction: Rectal intussusception is the telescoping of the rectal wall into the rectal lumen which can occur to varying degrees. Depending on the extent, it can give rise to a variety of clinical manifestations ranging from constipation to faecal incontinence. The aetiological factors are complex and a rational treatment strategy can only be devised after appropriate investigations. Without this, patients tend to have persistent symptoms resulting in considerable decrease in their quality of life.

Methods: Literature searches were carried out on databases such as Pubmed, MEDLINE, CINAHL and Google Scholar using the terms 'rectal intussusception,' 'obstructive defecation syndrome,' 'faecal incontinence,' 'rectal prolapse,' 'surgical,' 'management' and 'pelvic floor.' The bibliographies were also searched for relevant articles and back chaining was performed to obtain further articles of importance.

Discussion: In this article, the pathophysiology, diagnosis and management of rectal intussusception is reviewed. After reading this article, the reader would have a good understanding of the complex interplay of factors that result in rectal intussusception and how the various degrees of severity can give rise to different clinical syndromes.

Conclusion: Rectal intussusception is a disorder with a complex aetiology. Optimal treatment can only be achieved with a thorough history, appropriate investigations and a good understanding of the underlying pathophysiological mechanisms.

Chapter 3 – The Japanese Society of Emergency Pediatrics published clinical guidelines for the management of intussusceptions in children in 2012. The guidelines aimed to guide clinicians in order to diagnose intussusceptions as early as possible, to initiate appropriate treatment promptly, and to protect intussuscepted children from bowel necrosis, perforation, and shock. Three criteria of "diagnostic criteria," "severity assessment criteria," and "criteria for patient transfer" were proposed for these purposes.

The guidelines consisted of 50 clinical questions and the answers. Grades of recommendation were added to the procedures on the basis of the strength of evidence levels. Barium was no longer recommended for enema reduction, because the patient becomes severely ill once perforation occurs. Use of other contrast media such as water-soluble contrast, normal saline, or air was recommended under either fluoroscopic or sonographic guidance.

Liquid enema using water-soluble contrast was suggested to start with caution at a pressure of 100 cmH_2O and gradually increased to a maximum limit of 120 cmH_2O. With gas reduction, gas was suggested to inflate into the rectum at the initial pressure of 80 mmHg which may be increased up to 120 mmHg. Infants under 6 months of age were warned for a higher risk of perforation. The starting pressure of liquid and gas enemas in infants under 6 months of age was suggested to suppressed as low as 80 cmH_2O and 60 mmHg respectively, with special caution in increasing the pressure. Delayed repeat enema was recommended for improvement of reduction success rate, if the initial enema partially reduced the intussusception and if the patient condition is stable.

Before publication of the guidelines, a survey of the current management of intussusception in Japan was performed in 2011. A postal questionnaire was sent to members of the Japanese Society of Emergency Pediatrics, and the response rate was 41%. The results are shown under the "current management in Japan" at the end of each section.

Chapter 4 – Intrauterine bowel intussusception is rare. Foetal intussusception can be responsible of intestinal gangrene and resorption of the intussuscepted portions of the bowel and intestinal atresia may result. Prenatal diagnosis is possible but difficult, the prenatal features remain unknown in 60% of the cases.

Postnatally, the newborn presents an acute neonatal occlusion with bilious vomiting and distended abdomen. The diagnosis is currently made during surgery for acute bowel obstruction.

There are few cases described that demonstrate the intrauterine intussusception as a cause of intestinal atresia. When intestinal atresia is discovered an attentive examination of the distal part of the atresia would assist the classification of atresia and help in the understanding of the mechanism of occurrence, and to determine if there is or not an antenatal intussusceptions.

Chapter 5 – Small bowel obstructions are one of the most common indications for surgical intervention for patients presenting to the Emergency Room in the United States. Causes for small bowel obstruction can be divided into several categories: Extraluminal, Intrinsic, and intraluminal causes. The most common cause for the occurrence of an obstruction is adhesions secondary to prior surgeries. Delayed treatment or non-response of an obstruction to medical therapy could potentially lead to perforation, sepsis and ultimately death. Intussusception, or telescoping of the intestine, is a more rare diagnosis, but the natural history is very similar to small bowel obstruction. Prompt diagnosis and initial empiric therapy are critical in the management of both conditions. Treatment for both of these processes is at first non-surgical, however worsening of the patients clinic horizon will ultimately necessitate surgical intervention. Historically, general surgeons would perform a laparotomy in order to access the bowel for adhesiolysis. In the last several decades with the advent and improvement of laparoscopic methods, there has been a paradigm shift to diagnostic and therapeutic laparoscopy which is now currently preferred by most academic surgeons. Recent literature shows that minimally invasive techniques are becoming the gold standard for most gastrointestinal surgical procedures, citing reduced length of stay and improved pain control with similar rates of success. In this book chapter, the authors examine the diagnosis, etiology, pathophysiology and treatment modalities for both small bowel obstruction and intussusception of the small bowel, focusing on minimally invasive surgical options. This is a compilation of the most up to date information on diagnosis and management as well as a review of the current literature regarding safety and efficacy of the least invasive surgical techniques.

Chapter 6 – infrequently occurs following construction of a gastrojejunostomy. The operations most commonly associated with this complication are gastrectomy with Billroth II or Roux-en-Y reconstruction, and pancreaticoduodenectomy with conventional loop or Roux-en-Y reconstruction. Etiology of afferent loop obstruction includes: (a) entrapment, compression and kinking by postoperative adhesions; (b) internal herniation, volvulus and intussusception; (c) scarring and stenosis due to ulceration at the gastrojejunostomy site and radiation enteritis; (d) cancer recurrence; (e) enteroliths, bezoars and foreign bodies. Acute afferent loop obstruction is associated with complete obstruction of the afferent loop and represents a surgical emergency, whereas chronic afferent loop obstruction is associated with partial obstruction. Abdominal MDCT is the diagnostic study of choice. CT appearance of the obstructed afferent loop is a C-shaped, fluid-filled tubular mass located in the midline between the abdominal aorta and the superior mesenteric artery with valvulae conniventes projecting into the lumen. The cornerstone of treatment is surgery. Surgery includes: (a) adhesiolysis and reconstruction for benign causes; (b) by-pass or excision and reconstruction for malignant causes. However, endoscopic and transhepatic or direct percutaneous interventions for enteral stent insertion have the principal role in the in the management of malignant and radiation-induced obstruction. Nevertheless, considerable limitations exist as a former Roux-en-Y reconstruction limits endoscopic access to the afferent loop and percutaneous approaches for enteric stenting and tube enterostomy have only been reported in the literature as isolated cases.

Chapter 7 – Small bowel obstruction (SBO) is a common complication typically caused by adhesions that form after abdominal surgery, in response to inflammation associated with post-surgical healing. Adhesion formation occurs in an estimated 50-100% of abdominal or pelvic surgery patients and is the most common etiology of SBO. In the United States, adhesion-related SBO is a major health care expenditure annually.

Treatment options for adhesive SBO range from supportive care, consisting of bowel rest and intravenous fluids, to surgical intervention. While the non-invasive treatment options are effective at treating the current obstructive episode, the underlying cause of the obstructions – adhesions -- is not addressed. Surgical intervention is effective in treating the adhesions causing the current obstruction; however, surgery is the primary cause of adhesion formation and, thus, patients with a history of adhesion formation are at risk for developing additional adhesions and subsequent obstructions requiring additional surgeries. There continues to be research -- with limited success -- into methods of adhesion formation reduction in surgical techniques, medications and adhesion barriers.

Manual physical therapy has been demonstrated to deform adhesions within the abdomen and pelvis, allowing the pelvic and abdominal tissues and to function more normally. The manipulation of soft tissues to generate systemic functional benefits is not a new concept. In the field of osteopathic manual therapy, skilled manipulation of the soft tissues has long been believed to affect biomechanical change in adhesions such that the involved tissues exhibit increased pliability and independence of mobility. The authors have demonstrated a high rate of success treating post-surgical adhesions that cause recurrent obstructions. Patients report long term benefits from treatment and improvements in overall quality of life. Treatment with manual physical therapy compared to standard treatments will be discussed in the context of recurrent small bowel obstructions.

Chapter 8 – Bowel obstructions in patients with primary or metastasized cancer within the abdomen and pelvis are common occurrences. These patients experience bowel obstructions due to two distinct etiologies, malignant or non-malignant. The malignant cause of bowel obstruction is a mass obstructing the bowel, while non-malignant obstructions are the result of adhesions disrupting normal bowel function. Adhesion formation in response to radiation, chemotherapy, surgery and other treatments for the malignancy occur in 50-100% of gynecological cancer patients.

Treatment options for bowel obstruction are limited regardless of etiology. Patients undergoing treatment for cancer or that are considered palliative are often not surgical candidates and treatment is supportive with the goal of decreasing symptoms and pain control. Supportive care is often effective in resolving the current obstruction; but, patients are often on restricted diets and experience a significantly decreased quality of life due to recurrent partial or total bowel obstructions.

There is a significant interest in non-invasive treatment options that improve quality of life for these patients. The authors have demonstrated efficacy of a manual physical therapy regimen in treating non-malignant bowel obstructions in both active cancer patients as well as those who are in remission and are experiencing bowel obstructions due to surgery and treatment of the malignancy. A literature review of traditional medical treatment options and the authors' experience in treating gynecological cancer patients with non-malignant bowel obstruction using manual physical therapy is presented.

In: Intussusception and Bowel Obstruction
Editor: Rosie Miller
ISBN: 978-1-63482-703-4

Chapter 1

Intussusception: Symptoms

T. Dionysis*[*], *MD, and P. Petropoulos, MD
Athens Children's Hospital 'Euroclinic',
Pediatric Surgery Department, Greece

Abstract

Intussusception is the most frequent cause of bowel obstruction in infants and toddlers. It is an acquired invagination of the proximal bowel (intussusceptum) into the distal bowel (intussuscipiens). The classic presentation is an infant or a young child with intermittent, crampy abdominal pain associated with 'currant jelly' stools and a palpable mass on physical examination, although this triad is seen in less than a fourth of children. Vomiting is seen in 80 per cent; this maybe an early reflex feature or bilious if complete obstruction has occurred. Infants present more often with vomiting than older children do (up to 45%). Bilious vomiting tends to be found in delayed cases of intussusception with SBO. Occasionally, infants will present to the admitting pediatrician with severe lethargy and features suggestive of meningitis. The absence of pain, however, does not rule out intussusceptions but may delay the diagnosis. It is important to know that about 15% of infants and children present without any obvious pain. These children are often pale and listless and appear quite ill. In this chapter, we develop the symptoms and clinical findings of the intussusception.

[*] Corresponding author: thdionysis@gmail.com.

Clinical presentation of intussusception consists of the classical quadrat of abdominal pain, vomiting, palpable abdominal mass, and rectal bleeding. The presentation of each varies in accordance of geographical, socioeconomic, or even era criteria.

The two common symptoms of intussusception are abdominal pain and vomiting.

Pain is often the only or the early starting symptom of the disease. It is described as colicky, intermittent, severe pain, which starts acutely and that lasts for a few minutes. After the episode, the child is quite and pale. The attack often ceases as suddenly as it started. The episodes become more prominent as time passes. It must be emphasized that there are cases of intussusception with no reported pain. This happens more often in older children.

A heterogeneous group is oncology patients. Especially, pediatric patients after Wilms operation may suffer from intussusception without pain. These intussusceptions are spontaneously reducible. Also, children with recurrent Burkitt's lymphoma may occur intussusception without pain.

Olivier Abbo et al. [3] presents an interesting case of 17-year-old girl who was in the 5th year of follow up after an osteogenic osteosarcoma of the femur. She was treated for his primary tumor with chemotherapy (AOST 0331 protocol) and amputation. Also, after that she required thoracotomy twice for lung metastasis and four courses of chemotherapy. This patient was admitted with mild abdominal pain and no vomiting. The CT-scan revealed an ileo-ileal intussusception.

Also, in places with difficulty in reaching medical facilities, and in developing countries, it is often underestimated from both the parents and the medical practitioners. With the absence or underestimation of pain, the time needed for the correct diagnosis doubles with the children presenting in a worst hypovolemic state, and with a much more prominent bowel ischemia. The absence of pain, however, does not rule out intussusception but may delay diagnosis.

Vomiting is the other main symptom of intussusception. It sometimes precedes pain or exists in the absence of it. It is more prominent in infants than in older children. Because there is usually a short history of gastroenteritis, the vomiting is sometimes mistaken for gastritis. Both Ravitch [15] and Young [16] wrote that not only did most countries have similar clinical pictures of intussusception, but they also found that vomiting was the most common initial symptom (44%), ahead of the classic abdominal pain. Bilious vomiting occurs due to bowel obstruction in later-diagnosed disease. Also, due to bilious vomiting, the child suffers from acidosis and hypovolemia.

The two classical signs are palpable abdominal mass and rectal bleeding. They occur in the same frequency.

The palpable abdominal mass is sausage-like in the right upper quadrant going along the transverse colon toward the epigastrium. It is often accompanied with absence of bowel movements in the right lower quadrant, something easily understood by the pathophysiology of the intussusception, signe de Dance. Dionysis et al. [1] describes a laparoscopically extracorporeal treatment of irreducible intussusceptions, which presented with Signe de Dance sign.

The sign is often misdiagnosed in the developed countries nowadays due to the extended use of the ultrasound from the early steps. On the other hand, it is even visible in late-diagnosed cases. As the disease progresses, it is possible for the "head" to protrude through the anus and can be mistaken for rectal prolapse. Torres et al. [6] describes cases of rectosigmoid intussusception in which sigmoid colon intussusception was diagnosed as rectal prolapse, preoperatively.

Very interesting is the study of Ameh et al. [7] for the rectal prolapsed intussusception in infants and associated high morbidity and mortality. In total amount of 17 children who treated for intussusception, 29% was presented with rectal prolapsed. The clinical findings were mainly protruding anal mass, diarrhea, and vomiting. Abdominal pain and passage of bloody stools occurred late. There was a delay in referral and treatment owing to misdiagnosis as rectal prolapse. Four of these five children died. It is very important to diagnose a rectal prolapsed of intussusception. If we perform a rectal examination in intussusception we find a gap between the 'head' of the protruded bowel and the rectal wall. This is most important differential diagnosis sign between rectal prolapsed and rectal prolapsed intussusception.

Also, an interesting study presents Ramachandran P et al. In his series, prolapsed intussusceptions occur in around 8% of patients. The interesting thing in this study is that the patients were admitted with rectal bleeding and abdomen mass. The duration of symptoms were less than 48 hours, and the air enema reduction was successful in 57%. Also, from this study, it was concluded that a high index of suspicion is necessary for diagnosis of rectal prolapsed intussusception.

Absence of the classical triad of intussusception i.e. palpable abdominal mass, colicky abdominal pain, and bleeding per rectum, present more often in rare cases of intussusception as cases of sigmoid-rectal intussusception. Singh RB et al., [8].

The classical description of the rectal bleeding is described as currant-jelly-like with a significant amount of blood in it. This is a result of bowel wall ischemia. In the late-stage disease the whole bowel wall may be necrotic, and the children may suffer from premortal peritonitis.

It is the most alarming of the signs and symptoms of intussusception, and the one that usually takes the child to the medical facility. Most medical practitioners are aware of the rectal bleeding and the abdominal pain, but it must be emphasized hereby that rectal bleeding is usually the last of the quadrant of the intussusception to occur. This is the reason that a rectal examination and a stool test for blood should always be performed.

A very interesting case report describes M Takeuchi et al., [9]. He describes a case report of intussusception, secondary anaphylactic reaction to salmon roe. The 2-year-old patient was admitted with abdominal pain following ingestion of salmon with dyspnea, wheezing, generalized urticarial, and stools containing jelly-like blood and mucus.

Yamamoto LG et al. [11] assessing the value of the term "currant jelly''. They analyze the value of the stools in intussusception according to the experience of the physician. They studied 107 children with intussusception. Fifty-six children presented with spontaneously grossly bloody stools. Thirty-five children had rectal examination results charted. Eight of these children had grossly bloody stools noted on rectal examination, 4 of which were determined on chart review to resemble currant jelly. The most common terms used in describing the grossly bloody stools were "bloody," "mucus," "red," and "diarrhea." So according to the above study, limited experience physicians will be more accurate in diagnosis of intussusception.

Additionally Losek et al. [13] answered the question about the diagnostic value of testing stool for occult blood in children with intussusception. Ninety-six children underwent a barium enema for suspected intussusception. In this study, fifty-seven of ninety-six children had intussusception and twenty-nine of them didn't have a history or signs of blood per rectum. Sixteen of these twenty-nine patients were tested for occult blood. Twelve of these had positive test for occult blood. In comparison, three (20%) of the children who did not have intussusception had stooled positive for occult blood. The writer concluded that stool with occult blood had a high association with intussusception. Others symptoms, except the palpated abdominal mass, are not significantly associated with intussusception. They concluded that when evaluating children with non-specific signs, stool testing for occult blood is suggested.

Another interesting group is the children with recurrent intussusception. Champoux et al. [12] studied the risk and features of recurrent intussusception. She and her collogues found that abdominal pain was revealed in 95% of the cases at first recurrence in intussusception and 100% during the second recurrence episode.

Also, vomiting was revealed in 48% of the cases during the first recurrence and 100% during the second episode.

Only 5% of the patients had bloody stools during the first recurrence episode, and 50% during the second episode.

None of them were lethargic and only 29% had abdomenal mass during the first recurrence episode, and 25% during the second.

Furthermore, in this study the question is answered about the duration of the longest symptom before seeking medical attention. The 23 patients in the case group had a range from 16 hours to 767 days (25th percentile, 48 hours; median duration, 40 days; 75th percentile, 160 days) between the initial episode of intussusception and the first episode of recurrent intussusception. The seven patients with two episodes of RI had a range from 36 hours to 1,532 days (median duration, 264 days) between the first and second recurrences. In the three patients with three episodes of RI, the time from their second to their third recurrence was 20 hours, 21 days, and 71 days, respectively; the time from their initial episode to their third recurrence ranged from 141 to 465 days. When considering all 33 episodes of recurrent intussusception, in only three (9%) of the recurrences was the interval between one recurrence and the next greater than 1 year.

It is very important to keep in mind the symptoms of intussusception at atypical ages. PeyvasTeH et al. present their 11 years of experience of intussusception at atypical ages of children and adults. In this study, 36 cases with diagnosis of intussusception at atypical ages, < 6 mo or > 2 yr, were included. A sausage-shaped mass was found in 8 male and 6 female cases. Currant jelly stool was found in 8 males and 2 females. Distention was found in 9 males and no females. Fever was detected in 9 male cases and 5 female cases. Also, from 25 male cases, 14 cases had anemia. From 11 female cases, only 4 had anemia.

The most frequent symptoms in the male group was abdominal pain (84%) and vomiting (64%). Less frequent symptoms were anorexia, restlessness, and diarrhea. All patients < 6 months had restlessness. In the female group, the most frequent symptom was abdominal pain and vomiting.

Hemodynamic instability with intravascular volume depletion may occur in children with intussusception. Tachycardia and decreased capillary return should prompt active resuscitation, Spitz et al. [14]. Stabilization of the children should be the main goal. Any effort of diagnosis or therapy should be postponed until the child recovers from the shock.

Ailie Lochhead et al. [2] found that most children were brought in with a history of abdominal pain and or crying (> 95%); 66% had vomiting, 28% had fever at presentation, and 27% had a history of blood in stools.

Mandeville et al. [5] studied the clinical findings of intussusception. At presentation patients were stratified by age 1 year or younger, 1 to 3 years of age, and older than 3 years. There were 16 children older than 5 years (mean age, 117 months), and 9 were female. Overall, the most common clinical findings were abdominal pain, emesis, and guaiac positive or grossly bloody stools. Emesis and guaiac-positive or grossly bloody stools were more common in patients younger than 12 months compared with older children, with greater than 80% of the patients exhibiting these findings. Irritability, bilious emesis, and lethargy were also more common in patients younger than 12 months, whereas abdominal pain and abdominal tenderness were more common in patients older than 1 year.

James Jiang et al. [4] did a literature review for intussusception. He identified 82 studies from nearly all around the world, and he reported 44.454 cases of intussusception. This is the largest review study in the world. He found that the mean age of intussusception is 5-7 months old, and the incidence is 74/100,000 in infants under one year old. The proportion of children with intussusception who died after presenting to the hospital was substantially higher in Africa.

At the end, intussusception can occur in all ages but is more frequent from 3 months old until 2 years of age. The absence of pain or vomiting cannot exclude intussusception. Good medical history, good physical examinations, and good diagnostic tests may be life saving for a child with intussusception. Early recognition of the signs of intussusception may lead the physician to early successful treatment of this acute condition of infants and children.

If the diagnosis of intussusception is suspected, abdomen ultrasound is the first line for investigation and additional for therapy.

References

[1] Dionysis T. et al. Laparoscopic-Assisted Extracorporeal Surgery for an Irreducible Intussusception in a Child. *Hellenic Journal of Surgery* 2013; 85: 2.

[2] Lochhead et al. *Clinical Pediatrics* 52(11) 1029 –1033.

[3] Abbo et al. World Journal of Surgical Oncology 2013, 11:188.

[4] Jiang et al. *Global Intussusception Review.* July 2013 | Volume 8 | Issue 7 | e68482.

[5] Mandeville et al. *Pediatric Emergency Care.* Volume 28, Number 9, September 2012.

[6] Torres et al. *The American Surgeon,* Volume 76, Number 7, July 2010, pp. 718-720(3).

[7] Ameh et al. Transanal protrusion of intussusception in infants is associated with high morbidity and mortality. *Ann Trop Paediatr.* 2008 Dec;28(4):287-92. doi: 10.1179/146532808X375459.

[8] Singh RB et al. *Indian J Gastroenterol.* 1995 Apr;14(2):75.

[9] Takeuchi et al. *Pediatrics International.* February 2013.doi: 10.1111 /ped.12168.

[10] PeyvasTeH et al. Intussuception at atypical ages in children and adults – 11 years experiences. Przeglad chirurgiczny 10.2478/v10035-011-0047-z 2011, 83, 6, 304–309.

[11] Yamamoto LG et al. Stool appearance in intussusception: assessing the value of the term "currant jelly." *Am J Emerg Med.* 1997 May; 15 (3) :293-8.

[12] Champoux et al. Recurrent Intussusception.Risks and Features. *Arch Pediatr Adolesc Med.* 1994;148:474-478.

[13] Losek et al. Intussusception and the diagnostic value of testing stool for occult blood. *The American Journal of Emergency Medicine Volume* 9, Issue 1, Pages 1–3, January 1991.

[14] Spitz et al. Intussusception. Operative Pediatric Surgery. 7th Edition. Florida, *Year Book, 2013*, p469.

[15] Ravitch et al. Intussusception. In Welsch KJ. Randolph JG, Ravitch MM, et al. *Pediatric Surgery,* 4th edition, Chicago, *Year Book* 1986, p868

[16] Young DG:Intussusception. In O'Neil JA Jr, Rowe MI, Grosfeld JL, et al. (eds): *Pediatric Surgery,* 3rd edition. Chicago, *Year Book,* 1998, p1185.

In: Intussusception and Bowel Obstruction
Editor: Rosie Miller
ISBN: 978-1-63482-703-4

Chapter 2

Rectal Intussusception and Its Clinical Spectrum

Sanjay Harrison[1] and Harrison Benziger[2]
[1]Northern Deanery, Newcastle, UK
[2]Queen Elizabeth the Queen Mother Hospital, Margate, UK

Abstract

Introduction: Rectal intussusception is the telescoping of the rectal wall into the rectal lumen which can occur to varying degrees. Depending on the extent, it can give rise to a variety of clinical manifestations ranging from constipation to faecal incontinence. The aetiological factors are complex and a rational treatment strategy can only be devised after appropriate investigations. Without this, patients tend to have persistent symptoms resulting in considerable decrease in their quality of life.

Methods: Literature searches were carried out on databases such as Pubmed, MEDLINE, CINAHL and Google Scholar using the terms 'rectal intussusception,' 'obstructive defecation syndrome,' 'faecal incontinence,' 'rectal prolapse,' 'surgical,' 'management' and 'pelvic floor.' The bibliographies were also searched for relevant articles and back chaining was performed to obtain further articles of importance.

Discussion: In this article, the pathophysiology, diagnosis and management of rectal intussusception is reviewed. After reading this article, the reader would have a good understanding of the complex interplay of factors that result in rectal intussusception and how the various degrees of severity can give rise to different clinical syndromes.

Conclusion: Rectal intussusception is a disorder with a complex aetiology. Optimal treatment can only be achieved with a thorough history, appropriate investigations and a good understanding of the underlying pathophysiological mechanisms.

Introduction

Pelvic floor disorders include a group of disorders that are making their way to the forefront of gynaecology, urology and colorectal surgery. These disorders are increasingly common and very often result in a significant decrease in the quality of life of the affected individual [1]. The pelvic floor has three main compartments which includes the colorectal compartment, the gynaecological compartment and the urological compartment which all in turn act in a coordinated manner to maintain the structural and functional integrity of the pelvic floor. Anatomical and physiological alterations that occur to either a combination of these compartments or in isolation result in the various symptoms that eventually brings the patient to the attention of the pelvic floor specialist. In clinical practice, it is very often the case that the patient presents to the pelvic floor clinic with a combination of compartmental abnormalities. This combination of multiple pathologies can pose diagnostic and therapeutic challenges to the clinician.

There has been increasing interest amongst colorectal surgeons in pelvic floor disorders over the last two decades. This has been accompanied by a concomitant improvement in radiological techniques. The observed increase in the prevalence of pelvic floor disorders has been driven partly by improved diagnosis due to increased interest and awareness among clinicians along with technological improvements in various imaging techniques [2]. As isolated compartmental pathologies are rare, optimal treatment of pelvic floor disorders requires a very close collaboration of specialists which draw from urology, gynaecology and colorectal surgery amongst others. It is also noted that in addition to the physical debilities caused by pelvic disorders, there are attendant psychological problems that result and even predispose to pelvic floor dysfunction. Other health care professionals that have a significant role in the management of these patients include, nurse specialists, anorectal physiologists, gastroenterologists and even psychologists. It is therefore apparent that the very multidisciplinary nature of pelvic floor disorders necessitates a wide clinical approach that transcends what are otherwise well circumscribed specialty barriers.

The most common pelvic disorder that a colorectal surgeon would encounter in his or her practice would be a prolapse of the rectum. This can either be in the acute setting which is usually seen in elderly patients, or in younger patients in varying degrees which can present as constipation and in certain cases even faecal incontinence. It is therefore of prime importance for the colorectal specialist to elicit a thorough history and perform an adequate physical examination to further inform and direct subsequent investigations. It is important to note that as a specialty, pelvic floor disorders is still in its infancy and clear cut guidelines are yet to be laid down with regards to the optimal management of many pelvic floor conditions. Part of the reason for this is that the complex interactions between the various components of the pelvic floor and how they bring about 'normal function' is yet to be completely elucidated. While the condition of a complete rectal prolapse or procidentia may not present too much of a clinical dilemma, the case of rectal intussusception is not so straight forward. The various degrees of rectal intussusception manifest differently in different individuals, and in these cases the clinician would need to be guided very much by the severity of the patient's symptoms.

Given the complexity of the underlying aetiology, the clinician would need a thorough understanding of the anatomy and physiology of the pelvic floor components to treat and investigate the patient optimally. The main objective of this article is to provide the clinician with that knowledge and to also provide an overview of the various investigations and management options for rectal intussusception. While rectal intussusception can present in varying degrees ranging from minor mucosal prolapse to overt and complete rectal prolapse, in this essay these different stages are treated as a continuous spectrum rather than different disorders. Such an approach does provide the clinician with an integrated and coherent understanding of the aetiology and pathophysiology of rectal intussusception.

Key to the successful treatment of a patient with a pelvic floor pathology is the requirement of a productive and harmonious interprofessional relationship between all the involved parties. This vital professional cooperation can be facilitated, achieved and sustained by a proper understanding of the dynamics of interprofessional team working. It is important to note that the psychological aspect of the condition must not be neglected as it does play a considerable part in influencing the patient's perception of the severity of their symptoms. Managing the patients' expectations therefore is an important part of the management process. This aspect of the management of pelvic floor disorders which relies very much on input from a multi disciplinary approach opens up an avenue where the tools of management theory can be used to great effect.

Epidemiology

The first case of rectal intussusception was described in 1873 by Allingham and since then, with the advancement of various imaging modalities, it has been recognised to be a cause of evacuatory difficulty [3]. According to one study, rectal intussusception has been reported to be as high as 40% in patients presenting with evacuatory dysfunction [4]. It must also be noted that rectal intussusception has also been reported to be present in up to 30% of asymptomatic individuals [5]. This highlights the need for the clinician to interpret the radiological findings in conjunction with the patient's symptoms and examination findings.

Epidemiologically, it is evident that complete rectal prolapse tends to present in the elderly implying a role for ageing in its aetiology. It is believed this is related to the gradual weakness of the pelvic floor acquired with advancing age [6]. Complete prolapse does occur in younger patients but the underlying or initiating pathology tends to be related to collagen disorders, neurological disease and sometimes even diarrhoeal diseases associated with parasitic infections [7]. The latter aetiology is more commonly seen in children and tends to occur between the ages of 1 and 3. There is a considerable female preponderance with males only accounting for around 10% of cases [8]. This observation is yet to be satisfactorily accounted for but may be due the presence of the male prostate which acts as an anchor for many pelvic structures. Other risk factors include previous surgery, increased intra abdominal pressure due to chronic straining, pelvic floor dyssnergy, cystic fibrosis and Hirschprungs disease [9].

An epidemiological study by Kairaluoma et at looked at the incidence of rectal prolapse among a cohort of Scandinavian patients and estimated it to be 2.5 per 10000 of the population [10]. The median age was 69 years with an age range of 21 to 91 years. The cohort was overwhelmingly female and accounted for 90% of the group. Constipation occurred in 72% and incontinence was reported in 64%. Interestingly, it was noted that psychiatric illness was reported in 15% of the group. It is unclear what psychiatric illness in particular and whether this is an etiological factor or if it is a confounding factor due to the generally advanced age of most patients.

Variations have been reported in the degree of discomfort and bother experienced by different ethnicities. Dunivan et al. conducted a retrospective review of five hundred and eighty eight patients and collected data in the form of completed Pelvic Organ Prolapse Distress Inventory (POPDI) subscale and ethnicity [11]. There were no differences between the various ethnic groups with regards to age, prior prolapse, sexual activity or incontinence surgery. Their results revealed that patients of Hispanic and Native American ethnicity with stage 2 prolapse showed a higher degree of symptom severity when compared with non Hispanic Caucasian women. There were no differences between the groups with stage 3 prolapse.

The epidemiology of rectal prolapse and other conditions associated with pelvic organ prolapse is still incompletely understood. A recent review by Chow et al. anticipates an increase in the demand for pelvic floor treatment which would mirror the increase in the ageing population [12]. They draw attention to the fact that efficient and appropriate allocation of limited resources would require a better understanding by the physician of the incidence, risk factors, prevalence, natural history, clinical implications and treatment options. Such knowledge would also help develop new strategies to treat and ameliorate the associated suffering of patients with this condition.

Anatomy

As with most surgical conditions, a thorough understanding and appreciation of the diagnostic approach and management of rectal intussusception can be better obtained with a good knowledge of the underlying anatomy. The pelvic floor, which can be broadly divided into three main compartments on a functional basis, is comprised of the urological compartment, the gynaecological compartment and the colorectal compartment [13]. In this article, we would be focussing predominantly on the colorectal compartment as it is abnormalities in this compartment that can manifest clinically as a rectal prolapse of varying degrees.

The perineum is the inferior most pole of the trunk and is comprised of a complex of anatomical structures that lie between the peritoneum of the inferior portion of the pelvis and the superficial skin. The perineum is roughly diamond shaped and is bound by the lines that run from the junction of the two pubic bones at the pubic symphysis to the ischial tuberosities posterolaterally. The posterior half of the perineum is bound by the lines that run from the ischial tuberosities to the coccyx posteriorly, thereby completing the diamond shaped space. The surface projection of the perineum varies considerably with the position of the thighs and is reduced when the thighs are adducted and widened when the thighs are abducted or flexed. In the female pelvis, the perineum is crossed anteriorly by the urethra and vagina and posteriorly by the rectum. In the male, it is crossed anteriorly by the urethra only and posteriorly by the rectum rendering a greater surface area in the male perineum. The structures between the perineum and skin lie in three distinct planes and constitute mainly muscles and fascia [14].

The pelvic diaphragm which forms part of the pelvic floor consists of two laminar muscles which arise from the pelvic walls, are directed posteriorly towards the coccyx and rectum and attach to the opposite pelvic walls. These two muscles which are called the levator ani and the ischiococcygeus muscles, are invested superiorly and inferiorly by the fasciae of the pelvic diaphragm. The levator ani muscles are attached anteriorly to the pubis and to the ischial spine posteriorly and form a funnel shaped structure with its apex at the puborectal sling. This muscle is also attached to the fascia of the obturator internus via a tendinous arcade which runs between the two points of bony attachment. The muscle fibres are directed inferoposteriorly and medially which subsequently attach to the perineal body on the posterior wall of the anorectal junction and on the anococcygeal raphe. Anatomists have subdivided the muscle into different parts depending on their attachments and the relations to pelvic viscera as the pubococcygeus, iliococcygeus and the puborectalis. However, from a functional point of view these muscles very often work as a single unit and therefore the clinical significance of the anatomical distinction is not relevant. The levator ani muscles with their attachments, separate the posterior anal hiatus from the anterior urogenital hiatus. The ischiococcygeus muscle arises from the end of the ischial spine and is attached laterally to the margins of the fifth sacral vertebra and coccyx [15].

The most caudal and medial portion of the levator ani muscle is the puborectal muscle and consists of a superior and inferior lamina. From its insertion at the pubis, the inferior portion courses backwards to join the contralateral muscle just behind the anorectal junction, thereby forming a sling which anchors the junction to the pubis and determines the perineal flexure. The junction is anchored posteriorly by the anococcygeal ligaments to the coccyx. The medial fibres of the muscle course in a descending longitudinal manner and juxtapose with the longitudinal smooth muscular layer of the anal wall, interposing between the external and internal sphincters. The lateral fibres of the muscle have a predominantly antero-posterior course without as much a longitudinal descent [16].

The anal canal which on average is 4cm long begins at the anorectal junction and has a postero-inferior direction and is related to the perineal body anteriorly, the anococcygeal ligament posteriorly and the ischiorectal fossa laterally. The sphincteric muscles that surround the rectum cause the anal canal to take on the shape of an oval slit in the anteroposterior direction rather than a circular canal. The anal canal has three distinct portions which differ predominantly in the nature of the lining mucosa. The first portion which is 15mm long and begins at the anorectal junction and terminating at the dentate line is lined with stratified cubic epithelium. There are six to ten anal columns which contain terminations of the superior rectal vessels. The lower ends of these columns are joined by mucosal folds which are known as the anal valves. Between these lie small recesses also known as anal sinuses. The dentate line is the junction in the anal canal between its endodermal and ectodermal portions. The second portion which is also 15mm long is known as the transition zone and is lined by non keratinsed stratified squamous epithelium that contains numerous nerve endings but lacks sweat and sebaceous glands or hair follicles. This portion extends down to the line of Hilton which marks the boundary of the intersphincteric groove. The third part which is 10mm long extends from the line of Hilton and is continuous with the skin. The walls of the anal canal are surrounded by the puborectal muscle and the complex of internal and external sphincters [17].

The rectum, which forms the terminal portion of the large bowel is around 15cm long, is physiologically and anatomically quite distinct. Its physiological and anatomical integrity are essential in maintaining normal bowel function and aberrations in either or both of these aspects have been implicated in the pathophysiology of various pelvic floor disorders. It is continuous with the sigmoid colon at the level of the third sacral vertebra and descends down to the pelvic diaphragm in two distinct curves. The first is the sacral flexure of the rectum which lies along the sacrococcygeal concavity and the second is the perineal flexure at which point it crosses the pelvic diaphragm forming the anorectal junction. Two wide muscular bands are formed by the blending of the taenia above the rectosigmoid junction on the posterior and anterior aspects of the rectal wall. The upper third of the rectum is covered with peritoneum on the anterior and lateral aspects whereas the middle third only has a peritoneal covering on its anterior aspect. The reflection of the peritoneum in males superiorly onto the bladder forms the rectovesical pouch. In females, the peritoneum is reflected superiorly onto the posterior vaginal wall which forms the rectouterine pouch, otherwise known as the pouch of Douglas [18].

The rectovaginal septum is clinically very important particularly with respect to the operative management of rectal intussusception. Laparoscopic ventral mesh rectopexy which is now becoming increasingly popular as the operation of choice. The rectovaginal septum lies in an oblique orientation in the coronal plane next to the posterior vaginal wall. It is composed primarily of collagen, elastic fibres, smooth muscle cells and nerve fibres that originate from the autonomic inferior hypogastric plexus with a variable number of small blood vessels. Various histological and morphometric studies have evaluated the rectovaginal septum in transverse sections at three main levels ie the cranial (level I), middle (level II) and caudal levels (level III). The rectovaginal septum is thicker at levels I and III when compared to level II which gives it an hourglass shape and in the frontal plane there is a flattened central portion. The rectovaginal septum plays a crucial role in connecting the perineal body with the overlying endopelvic fascia. Given its position and relations, it may also play a crucial role in modulating pelvic wall musculature tone during endorectal pressure variations [19].

Pathophysiology

Procidentia or complete rectal prolapse is defined as a circumferential full thickness intussusception of the rectal wall beyond the distal end of the anal canal. The precise cause of rectal prolapse is yet to be completely elucidated and it is unlikely to be due to a single factor. Given the complexity of the pelvic floor and the inter relationships between the various components, it is likely that rectal prolapse and indeed, most pelvic floor disorders have a mulitfactorial aetiology. There is still considerable debate as to whether a complete rectal prolapse is the result of a worsening degree of internal rectal intussusception over a period of time or if it is similar to a kind of sliding hernia as it has been found in association with a diastasis of the levator ani, redundant sigmoid colon, loss of the posterior anchoring of the rectum and loss of the ano rectal angle [20]. It is noteworthy that similar manometric profiles have been noted in recto anal intussusception, rectal prolapse and in the solitary rectal ulcer syndrome.

Initial rectal intussusception tends to start at a median age of 44 years with the intussuception confined to within the rectum. In conjunction with chronic straining which occurs as a result of pelvic floor dyssynergy, the intussusception is believed to progress in extent which eventually presents as a complete rectal prolapse with a peak incidence between the ages of 70 and 89

[21]. Pelvic floor dyssnergy usually manifests as impaired evacuation which often precedes the development of a complete procidentia. The chronic straining that occurs results in vector force lines and increased intra abdominal pressures directed into the pouch of Douglas. This forces the anterior rectal wall to intussuscept which acts as the initiating event.

Anatomical findings have demonstrated that the perineal body is the point where the fibres from the perineal muscles decussate and cross the midline; an arrangement that allows simultaneous contraction of both sides of the muscles. This has the effect of shortening and broadening the central tendon and elevating the perineal muscles. This thereby acts as a perineal support against the increased intra abdominal and pelvic pressure, preventing perineal descent. Widening of the hiatus of the levator muscles exposes the perineal muscles to the increased pressures experienced during chronic straining and predisposes to further perineal descent [22].

Age also plays a significant part in the pathophysiology of rectal intussusception and it is known that the structural integrity and function of the perineum does decline with advancing age. Additionally, anorectal sensorimotor function which is assessed by the quality of anal squeeze and resting pressures, rectal compliance and rectal sensation are also known to decline. Perineal descent is noted to be more marked in older women indicating a degree of laxity which arises from impaired functioning of the muscles of the pelvic floor. This predisposes to the development of associated conditions such as perineal descent syndrome and obstructive defecation syndrome. Structural changes associated with the anchoring mechanism of the rectum have also been implicated in the pathophysiology of rectal prolapse and indeed many surgical approaches to its management are directed at correcting this in form of a rectopexy procedure. It is however unclear whether this is a result of the prolapse or a primary initiating factor in its aetiology [23].

The underlying support structure of the pelvic floor viscera, which consists of various muscles, ligaments and fascia, is complex and works in a co-operative and integrated manner. It is therefore unsurprising that defects in this system can lead to symptomatic rectal prolapse of varying degrees. Pelvic floor weakness has been demonstrated via defecographic and magnetic resonance imaging techniques and is noted to be characteristic of the perineal descent syndrome [24]. Histological and microstructural changes have also been demonstrated in the muscle fibres of the pelvic floor muscles that have undergone excessive stretching as a result of chronic straining [25]. Rectal prolapse has also been noted with a higher incidence in patients with connective tissue disorders such as Ehlers-Danlos syndrome and even in patients with cauda equine lesions or paraplegia. These are believed to be due to an underlying weakness of the pelvic floor. Rectal prolapse also occurs in paediatric patients who have undergone surgery for congenital anorectal malformations [26].

Presentation

The presenting complaint from the patient very much depends on the extent to which the prolapse is present. While it is most common in elderly female patients, it is important to note that it can occur at any age. The age of first presentation can also give an indication as to what the underlying pathology is and should therefore play a part in directing the clinician's subsequent investigations. With regards to a complete rectal prolapse, patients are usually acutely aware of when it happens and many patients are able to or attempt to reduce it themselves before seeking medical attention. Many times, spontaneous reduction of the prolapse does occur. Delayed presentation due to lack of patient awareness tends to occur in elderly patients with a degree of dementia and in very young children. Recurrent prolapse with delay in reduction can result in minor ulceration to the rectum which can result in the patient experiencing bleeding, mucus discharge and even tenesmus. Interestingly, many patients can also experience constipation and or faecal incontinence which precedes the development of complete prolapse [27]. A careful history would need to be taken to differentiate constipation that may be a result or manifestation of the obstructive defecation syndrome, from colonic slow transit or irritable bowel syndrome with a predominance of constipation.

The co-existence of various pelvic floor disorders with recto anal intussusception implies that a thorough history should also enquire about symptoms of related disorders. Evacuatory disorders which result in rectocoeles or enterocoeles are not uncommon and should therefore be actively enquired about in the history and looked for on physical examination. A patient reporting a history of having to digitate either per vagina or per rectum is suggestive of an underlying rectocoele and unless this is also satisfactorily addressed, symptomatic improvement following any surgical procedure is unlikely to be optimal. It is therefore of utmost importance that the clinician does not attribute the patients symptoms entirely to a rectal prolapse until any underlying functional problem has been addressed.

Another presentation of rectal intussusception maybe in the form of the solitary rectal ulcer syndrome. While the exact etiological mechanisms of this disorder have not been completely elucidated, it is believed to share a common aetiology with rectal intussusceptions [28]. Mucosal prolapse which is believed to be the progenitor pathology for rectal prolapse, leads to venous congestion, poor blood flow and oedema in the wall of the rectum which eventually results in ulceration. This is exacerbated by the continued and chronic ineffectual straining of the patient when evacuating their bowels. In addition to varying degrees of rectal prolapse, this condition can also present with rectal bleeding which is often described as bright red in colour, copious mucus discharge, prolonged and excessive straining, sensation of incomplete evacuation of bowels and perineal or abdominal discomfort. When occurring in the paediatric population, diarrhoea can also be present which can mimic the clinical picture of inflammatory bowel disease. Although, the commonest symptom of the solitary rectal ulcer syndrome is bright red rectal bleeding, it must also be noted that almost 26% of patients are asymptomatic and have a diagnosis made incidentally when being investigated for something else [29]. The diagnosis is made via endoscopic and histological examination of the rectum. Biopsies taken of the ulcerated area usually demonstrate abnormal glandular crypts, fibromuscular obliteration of the lamina propria and a muscularis mucosa which appears hypertrophied [30].

A certain proportion of patients who are found to have a degree of rectal intussusception do not present with any symptoms. This group has been estimated to constitute around 20% of radiologically diagnosed rectal intussusception cases [31]. Such patients tend to develop rectal prolapse without any preceding symptoms or rectal intussusception or associated structural or functional pathologies. It is not entirely clear why some patients remain asymptomatic and while others have more debilitating symptom burden despite a lesser degree of prolapse. One hypothesis is that this could be due to the latter group of patients having a higher degree of visceral hypersensitivity compared to the former [32]. This does occur in association with psychological problems and in many cases, the degree of pain experienced by these patients is attributed to the underlying psychological problem. While addressing this often neglected aspect of pelvic floor disorders, it must be remembered that unless no clear structural or functional abnormality has been found, the symptoms should not be labelled as 'psychological'.

Rarely, the underlying pathology of a rectal prolapse or intussusception may be a malignancy. Chen at al present a case of a 75 year old female patient who presented with a complete external prolapse [33]. Investigations revealed a recto sigmoid adenocarcinoma which had intussuscepted and then prolapsed through the anus. Yamazaki et al. also reported the case of a 76 year old female patient who presented with a sigmoid colon adenocarcinoma that prolapsed out through the anus [34]. The exact association between colorectal malignancy and rectal prolapse is not yet clear, but Yamazaki et al. propose that the prolapse was caused by the chronic constipation and was accelerated by the colon cancer. A similar case has been reported by Bounovas et al., [35]. Though these cases are rare, they do underline the importance of the need to investigate patients thoroughly in order to guide appropriate management. Any symptoms such as weight loss, anaemia, rectal bleeding or a significant family history should prompt endoscopic investigations as the first line prior to any further investigation of a possible benign pelvic floor disorder. This should also be the case in the elderly patient with a first presentation of rectal prolapse.

In the paediatric population, rectal prolapse can occur due to infectious diarrhoea. Again, a clue to the underlying pathology in such cases would be evident from the history. Khan et al. published a study in 2013 which looked at the clinical manifestations of shigellosis in 792 children under the age of 15 [36]. They reported that of the patients infected with Shigella dysenteriae type 1, 52% had a concomitant rectal prolapse. This was three times higher than patients without S. Dysenteriae type 1. As the mortality from infectious diarrhoea can be quite high in the pediatric population, prompt diagnosis with initiation of appropriate treatment is imperative.

Investigations

The first step in assessing the patient with symptoms of any degree of rectal intussusception or prolapse is a thorough history and examination followed by appropriate investigations which are guided by the findings of the former. Prroctoscopic and rigid sigmoidoscopic examination can be performed in the out patient clinic and can provide information as to whether the prolapse or intussusception has a low or high take off. During the physical examination, assessment can also be made of the extent of any perineal descent that would indicate a weak pelvic floor. It is not uncommon for an examination under anaesthetic of the rectum to be organised as part of the routine work up when radiological investigations are equivocal.

Once a clinical diagnosis of a rectal intussusception has been made, the patient is then subjected to appropriate radiological investigations to confirm and further characterise the underlying pathology. The most commonly used test to investigate rectal intussusception is contrast defecography and is now becoming the gold standard in many centres around the world [37]. This test requires the patient to ingest an oral contrast which opacifies the small bowel. Subsequently barium contrast is introduced into the vagina and rectum in turn and fluoroscopic images produced with the patient in differing positions. Further fluoroscopic images are taken with the patient straining and evacuating the rectum. Digital processing of the images allows measurements of the distances of pelvic organs and angles to be made. Other structural abnormalities of interest that can also be evaluated include rectocoeles and enterocoles. Rectocoeles which bulge anteriorly for more than 2 cm tend to be classified as pathological and would require intervention depending on the severity of symptoms.

There is much interest in the use of MRI defecography for evaluating patients with pelvic floor disorders. The lack of ionising radiation makes it particularly suitable for evaluating younger patients and it is also capable of providing good anatomical detail [38]. Sonography has also been used to evaluate the pelvic floor, and its distinct advantage over contrast defecography and MRI defecography is its ability to provide sufficiently detailed images of the anal canal including its mucosal and submucosal layers [39]. Pelvic defecography is another imaging modality that can be used to evaluate any structural abnormalities related to the pelvic floor, however its use is not widespread in day to day clinical practice as a good history can usually point to which pelvic compartment the predominant underlying abnormality is in [40]. Rectal prolapsed when treated as one end of the spectrum of rectal intussusceptions can be graded radiologically on a scale of I to V according to the Oxford Rectal Prolapse Grade [41]. This is illustrated in the table below. While there are numerous systems of grading that have been published, this system has the advantage of being simple and easily applicable and reproducible.

Despite the numerous advances made in the advancement of radiological modalities, the optimal imaging modality for evaluating the pelvic floor remains to be determined [42]. While each imaging modality does have its own advantages and disadvantages, in the absence of definitive evidence from large scale randomised controlled trials, a pragmatic approach would be appropriate in clinical practice. Contrast defecography is relatively cheap and easily available while MRI defecography exposes the patient to no radiation, however it is more expensive.

Grade of Rectal Prolapse	Radiological Characteristic
Grade I (high rectal)	Descends to proximal limit or rectocoele
Grade II (low rectal)	Descends to level of rectocoele
Grade III (high anal)	Descends onto sphincter/anal canal
Grade IV (low anal)	Descends into sphincter/anal canal
Grade V (complete external rectal prolapsed)	Protrudes beyond sphincters

The decision to subject the patient to any anorectal physiology testing depends on the history of the presenting complaint. In situations where an underlying neurological deficit or muscular disorder is suspected, it would be justified in arranging the appropriate physiological tests, however their use is not as commonly required as the radiological investigations mentioned above. In cases where the recto anal intussusception is advanced to a degree that it results in faecal incontinence, electromyography would be indicated to assess neuromuscular integrity once a sphincter lesion has been ruled out [43]. In such cases, endoanal ultrasonography is also indicated and provides complementary information that can affect clinical management. Chronic straining which very often occurs with the perineal descent syndrome can result in deficient functioning of the pudendal nerves. This is believed to be due to stretching of the nerve that occurs with the straining [44]. A similar decline in function of the pudendal nerve is also noted with advancing age. This can be evaluated with pudendal nerve terminal motor latency measurements. Vaccaro et al. conducted a study on 161 patients with chronic constipation and found that pudendal nerve deficiency was noted to be present unilaterally in 11.2% and bilaterally in 12.4% respectively [45]. Patients with paradoxical contractions of the puborectalis muscle were also found to have a significantly prolonged pudendal nerve terminal motor latency. The precise derangement patterns in the various neurophysiological parameters vary depending on whether the predominant symptom of the rectal intussusception is that of constipation or faecal incontinence.

Although electrophysiological tests can be done, currently there remains a lack of evidence as to the precise characterisation of the physiological derangements in patients with rectal intussusception [46]. Moreover, the clinical significance of pudendal nerve testing remains unclear with regards to its diagnostic and prognostic value as pudendal neuropathy has been reported in a large proportion of asymptomatic patients as well [47]. From a purely theoretical standpoint, one would expect these electrophysiological tests to play a significant role in the evaluation of the patient with rectal intussusception. However, most studies that have been published lack strict diagnostic criteria and vary largely with respect to methodology. This unfortunately makes combining results from these studies difficult and therefore conclusions remain equivocal [48]. The place of these tests in the work up of these patients remains subject to considerable amount of debate and at present they remain at best adjuncts to the main radiological investigations mentioned above and the clinician's physical examination of the patient.

Management

The decision to intervene in cases of rectal intussusception have to be based on and largely driven by the severity of symptoms. Managing the patient's expectations is also a crucial part of the process and the patient should be informed as to what extent symptoms may be improved with various treatments options. A useful strategy is to adopt a graded approach where the least invasive measures are instituted first leaving major surgical interventions as a last resort.

A trial of a conservative approach is worthwhile in most patients and includes laxative use, dietary advice and biofeedback and pelvic floor retraining. Most patients whose intussusception is driven predominantly by constipation and chronic straining should be trained to go to the toilet at a fixed time of the day or at times when the gastrocolic reflex is activated such as soon after a meal. Weight loss and physical activity is also reported to improve colonic motility and could also confer additional health benefits to the patient.

A trial of biofeedback should also be considered in patients who have evacuatory dysfunction presenting as their main symptom. This usually involves the use of several sensory modalities to re-train the muscles in the pelvic floor to act in a co-ordinated manner to achieve satisfactory bowel evacuation. This is particularly beneficial in patients who have a degree of anismus as well. The initial process involves educating the patient on the use of the appropriate position to aid defecation and to use associated muscles to augment the process. Sitting on the toilet with the feet supported off the floor usually with a low foot stool helps to open up the anorectal angle and prevent straining. Good short and long term results have been demonstrated in almost 60% of patients attending for biofeedback therapy with evacuatory dysfunction [49]. This is mainly reflected in the reduced laxative requirements and overall improvement in the patient's quality of life. These services are usually best delivered by a pelvic floor nurse specialist. The role of biofeedback in rectal intussusception is slightly unclear and that is primarily due to the paucity of studies that address this issue. Nevertheless, given the multifactorial aetiology of the condition, it would still be worthwhile having patients undergo a trial of biofeedback therapy to assess response. The current challenge in this area is being able to identify patients who would definitely benefit from this and thereby enable allocation of resources more efficiently.

At present, the role of sacral neuromodulation in the management of rectal intussusception is unclear [50]. This is largely due to the fact that in most studies, cases of constipation have been lumped together without much attention given to the underlying aetiology. It is therefore not clear that out of these studies how many patients had a degree of rectal intussusception that contributed to their evacuatory dysfunction. The role of sacral neuromodulation is more well defined in cases of faecal incontinence. Currently, sacral neuromodulation for constipation is not recommended by the National Institute of Clinical Excellence (NICE).

The general principle of surgical management involves eliminating the intussusception by fixing the rectum from above (rectopexy) or performing an excision procedure from the perineum. This principle has been applied in a variety of ways and has led to variety of operations being described. Initially, posterior rectopexy with or without a resection of the redundant bowel was advocated, however a Cochrane analysis revealed that such patients developed worsening constipation as a result of the operation [51]. This was put down to the fact that the posterior mobilisation of the rectum resulted in autonomic denervation. This procedure has now been largely abandoned due to the unacceptable side effects. Resection rectopexy has also gradually gone out of favour as the availability of an anastomosis free alternative in the form of a laparoscopic ventral mesh rectopexy meant that patients can avoid the risk of an anastomosis. Also, resection rectopexy does not address any concomitant middle compartment prolapse that is very often seen in patients with varying degrees of rectal intussusception or prolapse.

The laparoscopic ventral mesh rectopexy has now emerged as the operation of choice as it provides low recurrence rates of less than 5%, improvement in any co-existent faecal incontinence or constipation (ranging from 75% to 90%), only minor morbidity, short hospital stay of around 2 days and the opportunity to address middle compartment prolapse at the same time [52]. The improvement in bowel function is due to the autonomic nerve sparing nature of this procedure as only the ventral aspect of the rectum is mobilised. Perineal approaches for rectal prolapse such as the Altmeier's procedure and the Delorme's procedure have been evaluated extensively [53]. While it was initially believed that perineal approaches should be reserved for elderly and frail patients, new studies are beginning to show that in many cases the laparoscopic approach is safe and effective in the elderly population as well [54]. While a Delorme's procedure has the advantage of being repeatable should the need arise, like the Altmeier procedure it does have a fairly high recurrence rate varying between 5% and 25% [55].

Other procedures such the STARR and PPH procedure have been used in the treatment of patients with obstructive defecation syndrome which essentially excise the prolapsing focus of the rectal wall via a transanal approach. While these operations were initially taken up rather enthusiastically, subsequent reports of relatively high recurrence rates and serious complications such as pelvic sepsis requiring further major interventions have led to a more cautious uptake of these techniques. A major problem with the STARR procedure is the risk of damage to small bowel from an enterocoele or neighbouring structures which may go undiagnosed at the time of the procedure [56]. It is therefore essential that enterocoeles and any other structural abnormalities have been ruled out with the use of appropriate imaging prior to these operative interventions being attempted. The EXPRESS procedure is another operation designed for treating obstructive defecation syndrome and involves dissection of the rectovaginal septum via a perineal incision with lateral rectal wall mobilisation and suture fixation of the lower end of the recti muscles and a T shaped synthetic mesh in the rectovaginal septum [57]. Large randomised studies demonstrating the benefits of this procedure are lacking and this procedure is still only performed in a few centres only.

Conclusion

Rectal intussusception is a complex disorder with an equally complex aetiology. Its pathophysiology is intimately related to the complex functioning of the pelvic floor. It therefore becomes apparent that in order to treat this condition effectively, the clinician should have a thorough understanding of the underlying anatomy and physiology to better inform the subsequent investigations and management options. Due to its complex nature, a multidisciplinary approach is required when dealing with these patients as there very often is concomitant dysfunction of the adjoining pelvic compartments in addition to possible psychological problems which would also need to effectively addressed to achieve the optimal treatment. Cases should be discussed in the context of a multidisciplinary team meeting and decisions made on a consensus basis. With regards to investigating the symptomatology of the patient, there is still debate as to what the best modalities are, however it is unlikely that a single algorithm would be suitable for all patients and therefore subsequent tests would need to tailored to the patient's symptoms and their severity. This pragmatic approach also applies to the treatment options which should begin with conservative measures with increasing grades of invasiveness culminating in surgery if necessary.

References

[1] Fox, A; Tietze, PH; Ramakrishnan, K. – Anorectal conditions: rectal prolapse. *FP Essent*, 2014 Apr, 419, 28-34.

[2] Hatch, Q; Steele, SR. – Rectal prolapse and intussusception. *Gastroenterol Clin North Am*, 2013 Dec, 42(4), 837-61.

[3] Lunniss, PJ; Gladman, MA; Benninga, MA et al. – Pathophysiology of evacuation disorders. *Neurogastroenterol Motil*, 2009 Dec, 21 Suppl 2, 31-40.

[4] Weiss, EG; McLemore, EC. – Functional disorders: rectoanal intussusception. *Clin Colon Rectal Surg*, 2008 May, 21(2), 122-8.

[5] Dvorkin, LS; Gladman, MA; Epstein, et al. – Rectal intussusception in symptomatic patients is different from that in asymptomatic volunteers. *Br J Surg*, 2005, 92, 866-72.

[6] Poylin, V; Bensley, R; Nagle, D – Changing approaches to rectal prolapse repair in the elderly. *Gastroenterol Rep (Oxf)*, 2013 Nov, 1(3), 198-202.

[7] Sun, C; Hull, T; Ozuner, G. – Risk factors and clinical characteristics or rectal prolapse in young patients. *J Visc Surg*, 2014 Dec, 15(6), 425-9.

[8] Bordeianou, L; Hicks, CW; Kaiser, AM; et al. – Rectal prolapse: an overview of clinical features; diagnosis and patient specific management startegies. *J Gastrointesti Surg*, 2014 May, 18(5), 1059-69.

[9] Felt-Bersma, RJ; Tiersma, ES; Cuesta, MA. – Rectal prolapse, rectal intussusception, rectocele, solitary rectal ulcer syndrome and enterocele. *Gastroenterol Clin North Am*, 2008 Sep, 37(3), 645-68.
[10] Kairaluoma, MV; Kellokumpu, IH. – Epidemiologic aspects of complete rectal prolapse. *Scan J Surg*, 2005, 94, 207-10.
[11] Dunivan, GC; Cichowski, SB; Komesu, YM; et al. – Ethnicity and variations of pelvic organ prolapse bother. *Int Urogynecol J*, 2014 Jan, 25(1), 53-9.
[12] Chow, D; Rodriguez, LZ. – Epidemiology and prevalence of pelvic organ prolapse. *Curr Opin Urol*, 2013 Jul, 23(4), 293-8.
[13] Silva, WA; Karram, MM. – Anatomy and physiology of the pelvic floor. *Minerva Ginecol*, 2004 Aug, 56(4), 283-302.
[14] Barleben, A; Mills, S. – Anorectal anatomy and physiology. *Surg Clin North Am*, 2010 Feb, 90(1), 1-15.
[15] Raizada, V; Mittal, RK. – Pelvic floor anatomy and applied physiology. *Gastroenterol Clin North Am*, 2008 Sep, 37(3), 493-509.
[16] Guo, M; Li, D. – Pelvic floor images: anatomy of the levator ani muscle. *Dis Colon Rectum*, 2007 Oct, 50(10), 1647-55.
[17] Gordon, PH. – Anorectal anatomy and physiology. *Gastroenterol Clin North Am*, 2001 Mar, 30(1), 1-13.
[18] Charran, O; Muhleman, M; Shah, S; et al. – Ligaments of the rectum: anatomical and surgical considerations. *Am Surg*, 2014 Mar, 80(3), 275-83.
[19] Kleeman, SD; Westermann, C; Karram, MM. – Rectoceles and the anatomy of the posterior vaginal wall: revisited. *Am J Obstet Gynecol*, 2005 Dec, 193(6), 2050-5.
[20] Hoturas, A; Murphy, J; Boyle, DJ; et al. – Assessment of female patients with rectal intussusception and prolapse: is this a progressive spectrum of disease? *Dis Colon Rectum*, 2013 Jun, 56(6), 780-5.
[21] Thompson, JR; Chen, AH; Pettit, PD; et al. – Incidence of occult rectal prolapse in patients with clinical rectoceles and defecatory dysfunction. *Am J Obstet Gynecol*, 2002 Dec, 187(6), 1494-9.
[22] Rostaminia, G; White, DE; Quiroz, LH; et al. – Levator plate descent correlates with levator ani muscle deficiency. *Neurourol Urodyn*, 2015 Jan, 34(1), 55-9.
[23] Wang, GJ; Gao, CF. – The anatomy of the lateral ligaments of the rectum: a new perspective. *World J Surg*, 2011 Jan, 35(1), 227-8.

[24] Chang, J; Chung, SS. – An analysis of factors associated with increased perineal descent in women. *J Korean Soc Coloproctol*, 2012 Aug, 28(4), 195-200.
[25] Shafik, A; Ahmed, I; Shafik, AA; et al. – Effect of straining on perineal muscles and their role in perineal support: identification of the straining-perineal reflex. *J Surg Res*, 2003, 112, 162-7.
[26] Versteegh, HP; Sloots, CE; de Jong, JR; et al. – Early versus late reconstruction of cloacal malformations: the effects on postoperative complications and long term colorectal outcome. *J Pediatr Surg*, 2014 Apr, 49(4), 556-9.
[27] Dvorkin, LS; Knowles, CH; Scott, SM; et al. – Rectal intussusception, characterization of symptomatology. *Dis Colon Rectum*, 2005 Apr, 48(4), 824-31.
[28] Zhu, QC; Shen, RR; Qin, HL; et al. – Solitary rectal ulcer syndrome, clinical features; pathophysiology; diagnosis and treatment strategies. *World J Gastroenterol*, 2014 Jan 21, 20(3), 738-44.
[29] Edden, Y; Shih, SS; Wexner, SD. – Solitary rectal ulcer syndrome and stercoral ulcers. *Gastroenterol Clin North Am*, 2009 Sep, 38(3), 541-5.
[30] Al-Brahim, N; Al-Awadhi, N; Al, Enezi; et al. – Solitary rectal ulcer syndrome: a clinicopathological study of 13 cases. *Saudi J Gastroenterol*, 2009 Jul-Sep, 15(3), 188-92.
[31] Pomerri, F; Zuliani, M; Mazza, C; et al. – Defecographic measurements of rectal intussusception and prolapse in patients and in asymptomatic subjects. *AJR Am J Roentgenol*, 2001 Mar, 176(3), 641-5.
[32] Wijffels, NA; Angelucci, G; Ashrafi, A; et al. – Rectal hyposensitivity is uncommon and unlikely to be the central cause of obstructed defecation in patients with high grade internal rectal prolapse. *Neurogastroenterol Motil*, 2011 Feb, 23(2), 151-4.
[33] Chen, CW; Hsiao, CW; Wu, CC; et al. – Rectal prolapse as initial clinical manifestation of colon cancer. *Z Gastroenterol*, 2008 Apr, 46(4), 348-50.
[34] Yamazaki, T; Sakai, Y ; Sekine, Y; et al. – Sigmoid colon cancer presenting as complete rectal prolapse: report of a case. *Surg Today*, 1999, 29(3), 266-7.
[35] Buonovas, A; Polchronidis, Laftsidis P; et al. – Sigmoid colon cancer presenting as complete rectal prolapse. *Colorectal Dis*, 2007 Sep, 9(7), 665-6.
[36] Khan, WA; Griffiths, JK; Bennish, ML. – Gastrointestinal and extra intestinal manifestations of childhood shigellosis in a region where all

four species of Shigella are endemic. *PLoS One*, 2013 May 17, 8(5), e64097.

[37] Unger, CA; Weinstein, MM; Pretorius, DH; – Pelvic floor imaging. *Obstet Gynecol Clin North Am*, 2011 Mar, 38(1), 23-43.

[38] Piloni, V; Tosi, P; Vernelli, M. – MR defecography in obstructed defecation syndrome (ODS): technique; diagnostic criteria and grading. *Tech Coloproctol*, 2013 Oct, 17(5), 501-10.

[39] Brusciano, L; Limongelli, P; Pescatori, M; et al. – Ultrasonographic patterns in patients with obstructed defaecation. *Int J Colorectal Dis*, 2007 Aug, 22(8), 969-77.

[40] Faggian, A; Alabiso, ME; Serra, N; et al. – Entero-colpo-defecography vs supine entero-MRI: which one is the best tool in the differentiation of enterocele; elytrocele and edrocele? *J Biol Regul Homeost Agents*, 2013 Jul-Sep, 27(3), 861-8.

[41] Wijffels, NA; jones, OM; Cunningham, C; et al. – What are the symptoms of internal rectal prolapse? *Colorectal Dis*, 2013 Mar, 15(3), 368-73.

[42] Silva, AC; Maglinte, DD. – Pelvic floor disorders: what's the best test? *Abdom Imaging*, 2013 Dec, 38(6), 1391-408.

[43] Pereira, LC; Botelho, S; Marques, J; et al. – Electromyographic pelvic floor activity: is there impact during the female life cycle? *Neurourol Urodyn*, 2014 Dec 11 doi, 10.1002/nau22703.

[44] Engel, AF; Kamm, MA. – The acute effect of straining on pelvic floor neurological function. *Int J Colorectal Dis*, 1994 Apr, 9(1), 8-12.

[45] Vaccaro, CA; Cheong, DM; Wexner, SD; et al. – Role of pudendal nerve terminal latency assessment in constipated patients. *Dis Colon Rectum*, 1994, 37, 1250-4.

[46] Remes, –Troche, JM; Rao, SS. – Neurophysiological testing in anorectal disorders. *Expert Rev Gastroenterol Hepatol*, 2008 Jun, 2(3), 323-35.

[47] Ricciardi, R; Mellgren, AF; Madoff, RD; et al. – The utility of pudendal nerve terminal motor latencies in idiopathic incontinence. *Dis Colon Rectum*, 2006 Jun, 49(6), 852-7.

[48] Azpiroz, F; Enck, P; Whitehead, WE. – Anorectal functional testing: review of collective experience. *Am J Gastroenterol*, 2002 Feb, 97(2), 232-40.

[49] Kairaluoma, M; Raivio, P; Kupila, J; et al. – The role of biofeedback therapy in functional proctologic disorders. *Scand J Surg*, 2004, 93(3), 184-90.

[50] Ratto, C; Parello, A; Donisi, L; et al. – Sacral neuromodulation in the treatment of defecation disorders. *Acta Neurochir Suppl*, 2007, 97(Pt 1), 341-50.
[51] Bachoo, P; Brazzelli, M; Grant, A. – Surgery for complete rectal prolapse in adults. *Cochrane Database Syst Rev*, 2000, (2), CD001758.
[52] Gurland, B. – Ventral mesh rectopexy: is this the new standard for surgical treatment of pelvic organ prolapse? *Dis Colon Rectum*, 2014 Dec, 57(12), 1446-7.
[53] Shin, EJ. – Surgical treatment of rectal prolapse. *J Korean Soc Coloproctol*, 2011 Feb, 27(1), 5-12.
[54] Wijffels, N; Cunningham, C; Dixon, A; et al. – Laparoscopic ventral rectopexy for external prolapse is safe and effective in the elderly. Does this make perineal procedures obsolete? *Colorectal Dis*, 2011 May, 13(5), 561-6.
[55] Hotouras, A; Ribas, Y; Zakeri, S; et al. – A systematic review of the literature on the surgical management of recurrent rectal prolapse. *Colorectal Dis*, 2015 Mar 14, doi 10.1111/codi.12946.
[56] Pescatori, M; Gagliardi, G. – Postoperative complications after procedure for prolapsed haemorrhoids (PPH) and stapled transanal rectal resection (STARR) procedures. *Tech Coloproctol*, 2008 Mar, 12(1), 7-19.
[57] Williams, NS; Giordano, P; Dvorkin, LS; et al. – External pelvic rectal suspension (the Express procedure) for full thickness rectal prolapse: evolution of a new technique. *Dis Colon Rectum*, 2005 Feb, 48(2), 307-16.

In: Intussusception and Bowel Obstruction
Editor: Rosie Miller
ISBN: 978-1-63482-703-4

Chapter 3

Japanese Guidelines for Intussusceptions and Current Management

Yasuo Ito**, *MD, PhD
Division of Pediatric Surgery, International University of Health and Welfare, Atami Hospital, Japan

Abstract

The Japanese Society of Emergency Pediatrics published clinical guidelines for the management of intussusceptions in children in 2012. The guidelines aimed to guide clinicians in order to diagnose intussusceptions as early as possible, to initiate appropriate treatment promptly, and to protect intussuscepted children from bowel necrosis, perforation, and shock. Three criteria of "diagnostic criteria," "severity assessment criteria," and "criteria for patient transfer" were proposed for these purposes.

The guidelines consisted of 50 clinical questions and the answers. Grades of recommendation were added to the procedures on the basis of the strength of evidence levels. Barium was no longer recommended for enema reduction, because the patient becomes severely ill once perforation occurs. Use of other contrast media such as water-soluble

* Address: 13-1 Higashikaigancho, Atami, Shizuoka 413-0012, Japan, E-mail: yasuito@iuhw.ac.jp, Phone: +81-44-966-3664.

contrast, normal saline, or air was recommended under either fluoroscopic or sonographic guidance.

Liquid enema using water-soluble contrast was suggested to start with caution at a pressure of 100 cmH_2O and gradually increased to a maximum limit of 120 cmH_2O. With gas reduction, gas was suggested to inflate into the rectum at the initial pressure of 80 mmHg which may be increased up to 120 mmHg. Infants under 6 months of age were warned for a higher risk of perforation. The starting pressure of liquid and gas enemas in infants under 6 months of age was suggested to suppressed as low as 80 cmH_2O and 60 mmHg respectively, with special caution in increasing the pressure. Delayed repeat enema was recommended for improvement of reduction success rate, if the initial enema partially reduced the intussusception and if the patient condition is stable.

Before publication of the guidelines, a survey of the current management of intussusception in Japan was performed in 2011. A postal questionnaire was sent to members of the Japanese Society of Emergency Pediatrics, and the response rate was 41%. The results are shown under the "current management in Japan" at the end of each section.

Introduction

Intussusception is one of the most common causes of pediatric emergencies. Delay in diagnosis and treatment may result in bowel necrosis or even death of infants and children.

However, there had been no evidence-based guidelines for the management of intussusception in children neither in Japan nor in other countries until the Japanese Society of Emergency Pediatrics published clinical guidelines for the condition in 2012 [1, 2]. The guidelines were completed with the consensus of the Japan Pediatric Society, the Japanese Society of Pediatric Surgeons, and the Japanese Society of Pediatric Radiology, as well as the Japanese Society of Emergency Pediatrics.

The guidelines aimed to guide clinicians in order to diagnose intussusceptions as early as possible, to initiate appropriate treatment promptly, and to protect intussuscepted children from bowel necrosis, perforation, shock, and death.

The main recommendations of these guidelines are introduced as well as the current management of intussussception by a postal survey of the members of the Japanese Society of Emergency Pediatrics [3].

Methods of Formulatibg the Guidelines

The guidelines were prepared using the technique of evidence-based medicine. Literature was collected from PubMed (Ovid; 1966 to September 2009) and using the key words "intussusception" and "child" or "children," with limiting words of "human" and "English" and the internet version of the Japana Centra Revuo Medicina (Nippon Igaku Chuuou Zasshi; Ovid; 1983 to September 2009) with the equivalent key words of Japanese. Two thousands thirty three papers were collected (1275 English and 758 Japanese) including papers selected from references. The evidence level of each paper was rated in accordance with the Oxford Center for Evidence-Based Medicine Levels of Evidence (March 2009) [2].

The guidelines consisted of 50 clinical questions and the answers related to epidemiology, diagnosis, assessment of severity, and treatment. Grades of recommendation [2] were decide to the procedures of managements on the basis of the strength of evidence levels (Table 1) in principle, but social factors such as medical environment, cost performance, and the Japanese Health Insurance System were also considered.

Table 1. Grading system for rating recommendations [2]

Grade	Type of recommendation
A	Strong recommendation to perform this procedure There is good evidence to support its clinical effects.
B	Fair recommendation to perform this procedure There is fair evidence to support its clinical effects.
C1	Poor recommendation to perform this procedure The existing evidence is poor, but there is a possibility of favorable effects.
C2	Recommendation undetermined The existing evidence is poor or conflicting, and does not allow for making a clear recommendation.
D	Recommendation not to perform this procedure There is evidence to deny its usefulness, or to show its adverse effects.

Survey of Current Management in Japan

Before publication of the guidelines, a survey of the current management of intussusceptions [3] was performed in October 2011. A postal questionnaire was sent to 1783 members of the Japanese Society of Emergency Pediatrics, and 735 replies (response rate 41%) were received. Respondents were 542 pediatricians, 139 pediatric surgeons, 30 emergency room (ER) doctors, 1 general surgeon, and others (23), working in teaching hospitals (183), children's hospitals (86), district general hospitals (403), private clinic (58), and others (5). There was no radiologist member in the Society.

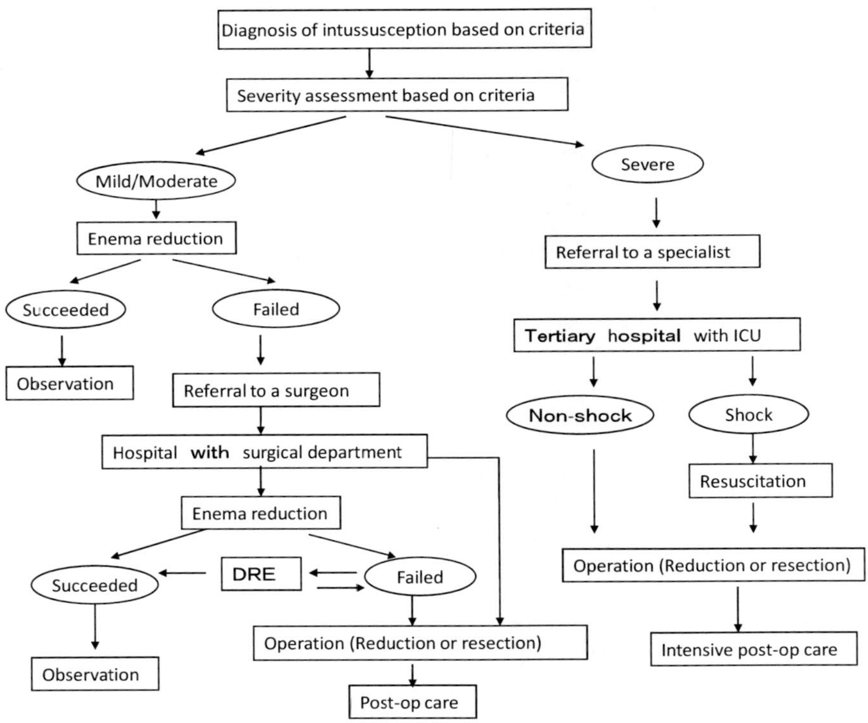

Figure 1. A flowchart for the management of intussusception in children [2] DRE: delayed repeat enema; ICU, Intensive care unit.

The draft of these guidelines had been presented in the annual meetings of the Japanese Society of Emergency Pediatrics since 2 years prior to the publication to reach a consensus, so that society members were thought to be influenced by the discussion to some extent at the time of the survey.

Flowchart for Management

A flowchart for the management of intussusception in children [2] is presented in Figure 1. The details of diagnostic criteria for early detection, severity criteria for severity assessment, and criteria for patient transfer for referral are described in each section. In these guidelines, the term "enema reduction" is used to represent hydrostatic and pneumatic reduction.

Incidence and Mortality in Japan

There are no national statistics regarding the incidence of intussusception in Japan. There are, however, a statistics of admitted intussusceptions registered at Diagnosis Procedure Combination / Per Diem Payment System (DPC/PDPS) of the Ministry of Health, Labour and Welfare [4]. During 6 months (from July to December) in 2010, enema reduction was undertaken in 2854 patients under 15 years old. Two hundred sixty intussusceptions were reduced by operation and 33 were operated otherwise.

The total number of intussusceptions for half a year will be 3147. But there is a possibility that all patients who underwent enema reduction did not necessarily had intussusceptions, because the diagnosis is made for the reimbursement of medical fees to hospitals. But the number of operated patients is assumed to be accurate. As the recent average reduction success rate in Japan is approximately 87% (87.3% by water-soluble contrast media, 90.2% by air, see Figure 5), total number of non-operatively reduced intussusceptions will be at about 2250 for half a year and 4500 for a year. As the number of live birth in 2010 in Japan was 1,071,000 [5], the incidence of intussusceptions was about 45 per annual 10,000 live birth. As the review of 14 Japanese papers showed that infants under 1 year old comprised 58.0% of 5279 intussusceptions [2], the annual incidence of 26 cases per 10,000 children under 1 year old was 6.7 times higher in comparison with 3.9 per 10,000 in New York States [6]. Japan had to wait until 2013 for the introduction of Rotavirus vaccination in infants. Mortality from intussusception is considered very rare in Japan, but there were 51 intussusception-associated autopsies of children younger than 14 years old reported to registry of the Japan Pathology Association between 1989 and 2008 [2, 7]. Forty of these deaths were infants younger than 1 year old. This is an average of at least 2.5 child or 2.0 infant deaths annually in Japan. There were 5 intussusception-related deaths for all ages registered at the DPC/PDPS [4] in 2010.

Standardized Diagnostic Criteria for Early Detection

The classic triad of abdominal pain, vomiting, and bloody stool were manifested in only 21-36% of cases at presentation [8-10]. In general, the earlier a child visits a clinic, the lesser the degree or severity of the symptoms. If the diagnosis is made promptly, most intussusceptions can be reduced successfully without operation. In addition, deaths from intussusceptions are avoidable. The diagnostic criteria were proposed in the guidelines [2] aiming at early detection of the condition and prompt initiation of the treatment (Table 2).

Criteria A consist of the three most specific symptoms and signs, and criteria B consist of less specific symptoms and signs. Definitive diagnosis is defined as characteristic findings of intussusceptions by imaging (criteria C). These diagnostic criteria are modifications of the case definition developed by the Brighton Collaboration Intussusceptions Working Group to investigate the association between vaccination and intussusceptions [11].

Abdominal pain including irritability is the most frequent presenting symptom of intussusceptions [8-10]. Intermittent and crampy pain is characteristic to this condition.

Bloody stool is also characteristic to intussusceptions, but is a late finding [8, 9]. Spontaneous passage of bloody stools is not commonly present at the initial stage of intussusceptions. Therefore diagnostic enema is helpful when intussusceptions is suspected. The presence of blood in stools increased from 40% to 97% [12] after diagnostic enema and from 53% to 71% by testing stools obtained by rectal examination for occult blood [13]. However negative bloody stools do not necessarily rule out the possibility of intussusceptions. Bloody stools were detectable only in 16% of cases with duration of symptoms less than 12 hours, and rectal bleeding was the primary sign in only 8% of cases [8].

Table 2. Diagnostic criteria for intussusception in children [2]

Criteria A

Abdominal pain or irritability
Bloody stool (including blood detected by enema)
Abdominal mass or distension

Criteria B

Vomiting
Pallor
Lethargy
Shock
Abnormal bowel gas pattern on plain abdominal radiograph

Criteria C

Characteristic image of intussusceptions by contrast enema, ultrasound, computed tomography or magnetic resonance imaging

"Suspicious diagnosis" is defined as when any of the following criteria are met:
One criterion A (abdominal pain or irritability) when it is intermittent
Two criteria A
One criterion A plus one criterion B
Three criteria B

"Definitive diagnosis": 'Suspicious diagnosis' plus one of the criteria C.

A tender "sausage-shaped" mass in the right upper quadrant of the abdomen is palpable in 30-85% of cases [8-10, 12, 14], depending upon the skill of the clinician. Emptiness of the ileocecal region (Dance sign) was observed in only 5% of cases, and was not diagnostic [8]. Abdominal distention appears at high frequency as a late sign after 24 hour duration [10].

Vomiting has a high incidence next to abdominal pain [8-10], but it lacks in sensitivity. The presence of the classic triad of abdominal pain, vomiting, and bloody stool is generally associated with long-standing duration of symptoms [8, 9]. Abdominal distension and fever occur more frequently in cases after 24 hours from the onset [10]. As a late sign, some infants present with profound listlessness and apathy [15]. Clinicians must also suspect intussusceptions in cases in which lethargy or septic shock is the first presenting symptom [14, 15].

There is no specific finding in blood tests to diagnose intussusception. However, if a patient is in severe condition due to bowel necrosis, leucocytosis is seen [16]. If the duration of symptoms is long, metabolic acidosis is expected. There is one report demonstrating that plasma C-reactive protein (CRP) was a useful marker to predict the clinical outcome of intussusceptions [17]. Abdominal radiographs are often unhelpful in diagnosing intussusception. Sargent, M,A.; et al. [18] reported limited agreement between three observers of radiographs and the diagnostic accuracy of abdominal radiographs was only 40% including equivocals. The best positive predictors of intussusception were opacity of soft tissue mass along the course of the colon and sparse large bowel gas in the right iliac fossa [18]. Lee, J.M.; et al. [19] reported radiolucencies in the soft tissue mass (crescent and target lucencies) as characteristic signs of intussusception on radiographs.

An ileocolic intussusception can be excluded by the presence of gas and feces in the cecum. Small bowel obstruction is a late sign and free peritoneal air is a contraindication of enema reduction [20].

Recommendations

1. If we include irritability and crying of unknown origin in infants in abdominal pain, abdominal pain is the most common clinical presentation, which is usually followed by refractory vomiting. Intussusception should be suspected at this early stage (recommendation A).
2. Confirmation of macroscopic bloody stools or occult blood by enema or rectal examination is helpful for diagnosis, when clinical symptoms are obscure (recommendation B).
3. A sausage-shaped mass is palpated in the right hypochondrium. The incidence of "Dance sign," emptiness of right lower quadrant, is low. Abdominal distension increases with time. Palpation of the abdomen is highly recommended (recommendation A).
4. Blood tests do not have a diagnostic value for intussusception, but they are useful to evaluate the general condition of the patients (recommendation B).

5. Plain abdominal radiographs have a limited diagnostic value, but they are useful to detect free peritoneal air or small bowel obstruction (recommendation B).

Current Management in Japan

According to the postal survey, diagnostic enema was performed almost always in 73.8% (537/728) of respondents, occasionally in 14.3% (104/728), and never in 11.9% (87/728).

Imaging for Definitive Diagnosis

Sonography is used as the modality of choice for screening intussusception at many institutions. It has great merit in that it requires no radiation. It has high sensitivity of almost 100% and specificity of 88-100% [21-23]. Intussusceptions can usually be found with sonography on the right side of the abdomen as a "target" [22], "doughnut" [22], or "crescent-in-doughnut" [24] sign in the transverse plane, and as "pseudokidney" sign [22] on longitudinal section.

Occasional false-positive examination includes any cause of bowel wall thickening, such as enterocolitis and hematoma. Therefore, scanning of both the transverse and the longitudinal plane is important for the diagnosis of intussusception [21, 23]. The disadvantage of sonography is that the accuracy of diagnosis depends on the experience of the operators, who may have insufficient training. If one does not have confidence in utilizing sonography, or sonography is not available in an emergency situation, contrast study is helpful to confirm the diagnosis [25]. Contrast enema has several merits, although it has the disadvantage of radiation exposure. The technique of contrast enema is easy to learn, well known to almost all clinicians, and is less likely to miss the diagnosis of intussusception than sonography.

Once the diagnosis of intussusceptions is made, the clinician can proceed to the reduction with the same modality [20].

Computed tomography (CT) has high resolution in the diagnosis of intussusceptions, but it is not practically used because of the larger dose of radiation required and the necessity for sedation. The use of CT should be reserved for delineation of small-bowel intussusceptions and/or a pathological lead point (PLP) in older children with atypical symptoms [26].

Recommendations

6. Sonography has nearly 100% sensitivity and specificity in diagnosis of intussusception, and is useful for screening the condition (recommendation A).
7. Sonography has priority for diagnosis, but if the diagnosis is uncertain, or when sonographic expertise is not available in an emergency situation, contrast enema study is necessary (recommendation A).
8. Considering radiation exposure, CT is not the first choice for diagnosis of intussusception. But it is useful when intussusception cannot be ruled out, or in rare cases of small-bowel intussusception (recommendation B).

Current Management in Japan

Sonography was selected for diagnosis almost always in 84% (615/730) of respondants, and fluoroscopy was preferred in only 9% (67/730). The rest used either of them depending on the situation (Figure 2).

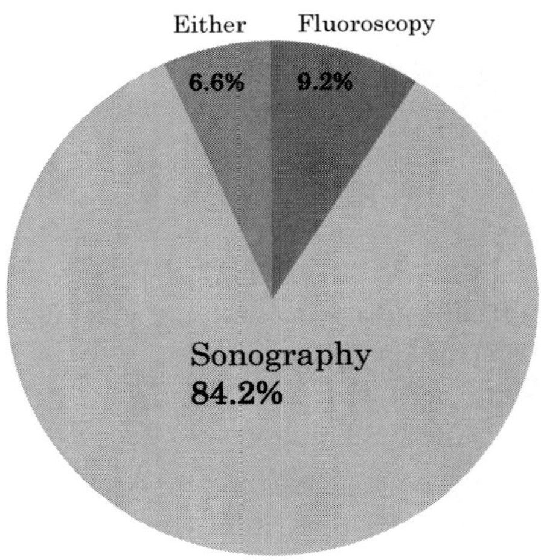

Figure 2. Replies to the question, "What modality do you use for diagnosis in suspected cases?" (n = 730).

Severity Assessment Criteria for Saving Severely Ill Patients

Intussusceptions is a strangulation obstruction, leading to bowel ischemia, necrosis, sepsis, and eventually death. There are a variety of degrees of severity from mild to severe in the pathophysiology of intussusceptions. The severity assessment criteria [2] were proposed in the guidelines aiming at selection of the appropriate procedures for diagnosis, treatment, or prompt referral to a tertiary hospital according to the severity of the intussusceptions (Table 3).

Table 3. Severity assessment criteria for intussusception in children [2]

Severe	Poor general condition or one of the following conditions indicating bowel necrosis 1) Septic shock 2) Peritonitis 3) Free peritoneal air on a plain abdominal radiograph
Moderate	Stable general condition, but one of the following conditions indicating possible ischemia of the bowel 1) Duration of symptoms beyond 48 h 2) Infants of 3 months of age and younger 3) The apex located beyond the splenic flexure 4) Ileoileocolic type 5) White blood cells > 20,000/μL, elevated CRP > 10mg/dL 6) Small bowel obstruction on a plain abdominal radiograph 7) Ultrasound findings of lack of blood flow, trapped fluid between intussuscepted bowl walls, and presence of pathological lead point
Mild	Stable general condition in which criteria of "severe" or "moderate" are excluded.

"Severe" intussusception is a state of poor general condition from its basic disease or suspected bowel necrosis. Poor general condition suggests gangrenous intussusceptions. Severe dehydration, septic shock, and signs of peritonitis are suggestive of a "severe" state of intussusception. After adequate resuscitation by intensive care, surgery is the treatment of choice. Contrast enema reduction is contraindicated, [27, 28] and sonography is preferable as a diagnostic modality.

"Moderate" intussusceptions is a state of stable general condition, but is accompanied by symptoms and signs of possible bowel ischemia. Enema reduction is not contraindicated but because of the possibility of perforation or unsuccessful reduction, cautious selections of contrast media, reducing pressure, reduction time, and reduction attempts are necessary.

Duration of symptoms of more than 48 hours was significantly correlated with failure of enema reduction and with a high rate of bowel resection [16]. The longer the duration of symptoms, the lower the likelihood of successful enema reduction and the higher the rate of bowel perforation [29]. However, a long duration of symptoms itself is not a contraindication for attempted enema reduction. For infants, age of 3 months and younger was associated with a low success rate of reduction [30], and younger age was a predictor of perforation [29]. The location of the apex has also been correlated with severity. Reduction success rate was low when the intussusception was encountered beyond the splenic flexure [31]. Successful enema reduction is less likely especially once the apex reaches the rectosigmoid region [32].

Among types of intussusceptions, the ileoileocolic type is also significantly correlated with low enema reduction rate [29, 33] and bowel necrosis [29].

Leucocytosis is more frequently seen in moderate-to-severe cases. In one study, the incidence of white blood cell count greater than 20,000/μL was significantly higher in the bowel-resection group compared with those of the operative-reduction group and the enema-reduction group [16]. Elevated CRP > 10mg/dL also reflects the degree of severity of the condition. The incidence of CRP > 10mg/dL was significantly higher in the bowel-resection group compared with those of the operative-reduction group and the enema-reduction group [17].

The presence of small-bowel obstruction is a risk factor for failure of enema reduction and for bowel resection [34], but it is not a contraindication to performing the enema. Free intraperitoneal air is said to be a contraindication for enema reduction, but there were no relevant cases documented in literature after 1966.

Absence of blood flow by Color Doppler sonography has been shown to be predictive of bowel necrosis and the need for bowel resection [35-37].

Detection of blood flow was associated with successful enema reduction, and lack of flow is suggestive of failure of enema reduction [36, 38, 39]. However, nonvisualization of blood flow by color Doppler sonography was not a contraindication for attempted air enema reduction [38]. These different results may be influenced by the sensitivity of the equipment used and the technique of the examiners.

Trapped peritoneal fluid between two limbs of the intussuscepted was also shown to be associated with a significantly lower reduction success rate and higher degree of bowel ischemia [40, 41]. Although trapped fluid is not a contraindication for attempting air enema reduction, vigorous, high-pressure enema reduction should not be attempted [40]. The presence of free intraperitoneal fluid in small or moderate amount does not predict a lower enema success rate, but a large amount of intraperitoneal fluid is predictive of surgery [21, 23]. The presence of a PLP is a risk factor for irreducible intussusceptions and surgery [9, 31, 42], but it does not necessarily mean that enema reduction is impossible [23].

There are no reports demonstrating a sufficient evidence level that discuss the correlation between CT findings and the severity of the intussusceptions. Sonography has priority in the assessment of severity. The use of CT should be reserved for special cases, in which sonography is of no use.

"Mild" intussusceptions is a state which does not fulfill the above mentioned conditions of "severe" or "moderate" intussusceptions. Patients with this condition are good candidates for enema reduction.

As predictors of bowel necrosis, duration of symptoms beyond 48 hours, ileoileocolic type, and lack of blood flow by color Doppler have been considered in previous clinical discussions. But none of these features, in isolation, is an absolute contraindication to enema reduction. However, a combination of these factors will significantly increase the risk of bowel necrosis, the possibility of bowel resection, and incidence of complications.

Recommendations

9. Shock, peritonitis, duration of symptoms, age, location of the apex, and invagination type do correlate with severity. Therefore, a detailed history of clinical symptoms and physical examination are important (recommendation A).
10. Leucocytosis of white blood cell counts > 20,000/μL and elevated CRP > 10mg/dL are often observed in moderate to severe

intussusceptions. White blood cell count and CRP are useful for severity assessment (recommendation B).

11. Free peritoneal air and small bowel obstruction on plain abdominal radiographs are useful for severity assessment (recommendation B).
12. Lack of blood flow, trapped fluid between intussuscepted bowl walls, and presence of PLP correlate with severity of intussusception. Sonography is useful for severity assessment (recommendation B).
13. Location of the apex and invagination type correlate with severity of intussusception. Contrast enema is useful for severity assessment (recommendation B).
14. There are a few case reports on CT findings demonstrating bowel necrosis. However, evidence levels are low and moreover there is a concern of radiation exposure in CT. CT is not useful for severity assessment (recommendation C2).

Criteria for Patient Transfer

Criteria for patient transfer [2] is proposed in the following "Recommendations."

Severely ill patients with peritonitis or in shock are contraindicated for enema reduction, and it is recommended to transfer these patients immediately to tertiary hospitals, including children's hospitals, where intensive preoperative care is possible and surgeons (ideally pediatric surgeons) are available. Enema reduction rate was higher, and hospital stay was shorter when patients were treated at children's hospitals in comparison with those treated at non-children's hospitals, owing to a positive volume-outcomes relationship [43, 44]. If an attempted enema reduction is a failure in mild-to-moderate cases, it is also necessary to refer these patients to a hospital where surgeons are available. Prompt transfer of patients is important for improvement in case management. Delay of transfer of more than 24 hours from a non-teaching hospital to a teaching hospital increased the incidence of operation significantly [43, 45].

Recommendations

15. Patients with severe intussusception should not undergo enema reduction, but should be transferred immediately to a tertiary hospital

where intensive care, including surgery, is possible (recommendation A).

16. Patients with moderate intussusceptions need careful attempt at enema reduction. If the attempt is in failure, the patient should be transferred to surgical facilities as soon as possible (recommendation A).
17. Patients with mild intussusception are good candidates for enema reduction. If the reduction fails, the patient should be transferred to surgical facilities as soon as possible (recommendation A).

Management for Non-Operaive Reduction

It is now generally accepted that non-operative reduction should be attempted in most patients with acute idiopathic intussusception. The apex of the intussusceptum is pushed back by hydrostatic or pneumatic enema. Different types of contrast media (including negative contrast of air) are used under the guidance of fluoroscopy or sonography. Various combinations of contrast media and monitoring modalities are possible.

Based on the reduction success rates published in the recent literature, one should aim to achieve at least an 85% success rate, and even as high as 95%. However, these rates will be influenced by the specific patient population one sees.

Fluid

In cases deemed moderate-to-severe by severity assessment, it is important to correct the child's hypovolemia and dehydration with adequate fluid replacement intravenously prior to surgery or enema reduction [27, 46, 47]. Dehydration is observed about in 50% of cases of intussusception [46].

In mild cases with good hydration, intravenous resuscitation is not necessary. However, placement of venous line is desired for safety to cope with complications that may arise during enema reduction.

Recommendations

18. In cases of severe and moderate intussusceptions, circulatory insufficiency and dehydration should be treated with extracellular fluid replacement (recommendation A).

19. In cases of mild dehydration, intravenous fluid is not necessarily required, but it is desirable to maintain the venous route to handle complications expected by enema reduction (recommendation B).

Current Management in Japan

Venous route was maintained almost always in 86.8% (592/682) of respondents, occasionally in 8.5% (58/682), and never in 4.7% (32/682) according to the postal survey.

Use of Anesthesia

Some authors, in the past, have recommended routine use of general anesthesia including gas [48], thiopenthal [49], and ketamine [50, 51], which they believed improved enema reduction rate. However no differences have been demonstrated in reduction rates between two groups with and without anesthesia [52, 53]. There are also papers recommending the use of general anesthesia in the second attempt in the operating room with improvement of reduction rates [54-56]. However, in these cases, improvement of reduction rates may possibly be attributed to the effect of delayed repeat enema (see the section of "delayed repeat enema"), not of general anesthesia.

Recommendation

20. There is no significant difference between enema reductions with and without general anesthesia. General anesthesia is not necessary for reduction (recommendation C2).

Current Management in Japan

General anesthesia for reduction was performed almost always in 17.5% (119/681) of respondents, occasionally in 17.5% (119/681), and never in 65.0% (443/681).

Use of Sedation and/or Antispasmodics

Various kinds of sedation such as diazepam [30, 50, 55, 57, 58], chloral hydrate [55, 59], pentazocine [60, 61], meperidine [15, 62], morphine sulfate

[15, 63, 64], etc. have been customarily used. There is a comparative study of analgesic premedication, which improved the reduction rate [62]. However the conclusion is of this study is questionable, because the reduction rate of the sedation group was 68%, while that of the non-sedation group was only 36%, which is extremely low. Therefore, there is little evidence to support or condemn the use of sedation. The use of sedation depends on the clinician's preference at present. Butylscopolamine (Buscopan®) has been used customarily as an antispasmodic agent, to irrigate the colon smoothly with contrast media [57, 65, 66]. However, there are no controlled studies evaluating its effectiveness. The use of Buscopan® is left to the clinician's preference at present. Glucagon has muscle relaxant effects as well as Buscopan®, and has been used for enema reduction. In earlier reports, the reduction rate was higher when Glucagon was used [60, 63]. However, more recent randomized controlled studies have shown that glucagon is of no benefit [67, 68]. The use of glucagon is not recommended as it is an expensive drug in comparison to Buscopan®, and health insurance in Japan may not cover the fee.

Recommendations

21. There are few papers discussing the effectiveness of sedation. The use of sedation is left to the physician's choice (recommendation C1).
22. There is no comparative study on the effectiveness of Buscopan® in enema reduction. The use of Buscopan® is left to the physician's preference (recommendation C1).
23. The effectiveness of glucagon in the improvement of reduction rate is inconsistent. Glucagon is not recommended for reduction (recommendation C2).

Current Management in Japan

Sedation and/or antispasmodics were used almost always in 21.0% (145/674) of respondents, occasionally in 15.9% (107/674), and never in 62.6% (422/674).

Selection of Imazging

There are many reports of enema reduction under sonography [33, 55, 61, 69-78] since Bolia's report [79] in 1985. The greatest advantage of sonography is that it does not involve radiation exposure to children, and therefore reduction can be attempted repeatedly without concern for time [55]. The modality of sonography has another advantage in that it is able to detect PLPs on reduction such as Meckel diverticulum or duplication cysts [80, 81]. The main disadvantage of sonography is the need for training of a clinician, because it is an extremely operator-dependent modality [70, 81].

There is no study on the direct comparison of reduction with fluoroscopy versus reduction with sonography, Considering the differences of medical environments and expertise of clinicians, the choice of either fluoroscopy or sonography depends on a clinician's favor.

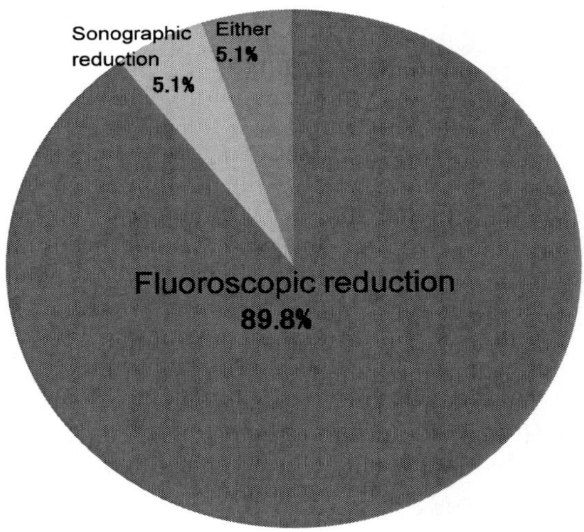

Figure 3. Replies to the question, "What modality do you use for non-operative reduction?" (n = 683).

Current Management in Japan

Fluoroscopic reduction was preferred in 89.8% (613/683) of respondents and sonographic reduction was selected in only 5% (35/683). The rest used either of them depending on the situation (Figure 3).

Selection of Contrast Media

After Ravitch's report [82] in 1948, the use of barium for enema reduction has become the definitive non-operative management throughout the world. However, the major disadvantage of barium enema reduction is the complication of barium peritonitis when perforation occurs during the enema [83-87].

Barium spilled into the abdominal cavity and mixed with feces cannot be removed completely. Barium adhered to the peritoneum and omentum remains radiologically for years and can cause intestinal obstruction later. Once perforation has occurred, patients with barium enema have been shown to require bowel resection more often, longer hospital stays, and increased morbidity rates compared to those with air [84, 88] or water-soluble contrast enema [87, 88]. Because of this risk, water-soluble iodinated contrast media such as diatrizoate meglumine (Gastrografin®) [85, 88 -91] or air [29, 46, 47, 49, 50, 59, 64] is preferred over barium as an alternative contrast media for enema reduction under fluoroscopy.

The advantage of the use of the barium enema reduction technique has been claimed to be its clear delineation of the reducing process of intussusception, but water-soluble agents diluted to iso-osmolar concentrations still allow appropriate anatomical delineation under fluoroscopy [85, 91]. Water-soluble iodinated contrast media is recommended instead of barium if one chooses hydrostatic reduction under fluoroscopic guidance. On the other hand, air is preferred outside of Japan, because it is considered cheaper and safer when perforation occurs. The disadvantage of the air enema technique under fluoroscopy is that the delineation of the intussusception image is less clear, and clinicians who are accustomed to positive contrast media may need to get used to it. Especially, it may be more difficult to visualize both the intussusception and reduction in patients with marked amounts of gas in the small bowel [50]. As for the contrast media under sonographic guidance, there are several series studies that have achieved equally high reduction rates using air [38, 41, 71, 73, 75, 76] or liquid [33, 55, 61, 69, 70, 72, 74], but no comparative study of air and liquid has been carried out. Either air or normal saline can be used according to the preference of the physician.

Recommendtion

24. Barium has traditionally been used as a contrast media, which most physicians are accustomed to. However, once perforation occurs

during the enema, the patient becomes severely ill. Barium is no longer recommended (recommendation D). Use of contrast media other than barium is recommended.

Current Management in Japan

Gastrografin® was preferred for fluoroscopic reduction in 67% (433) over air 23% (150) of 646 respondents. Barium which is not recommended in the guidelines any more was used only in 6% (40/646) (Figure 4). For sonographic reduction, normal saline was preferred in 73% (49) over air 15%(19) of 67 respondents.

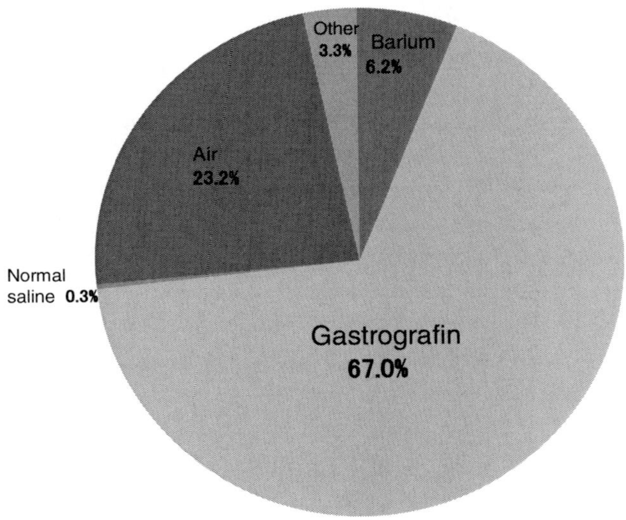

Figure 4. Replies to the question, "What contrast media do you use for fluoroscopic reduction?" (n = 646).

Comparison of Reduction Success Rate between Japan and Other Countries

Surveys [92-94] of pediatric radiology departments in North America and Europe have shown a trend among pediatric radiologists to change from hydrostatic reduction to pneumatic reduction techniques under either fluoroscopy or sonography. This change may be due to the lower reduction success rate in barium than in air or oxygen in comparative studies (53-85%

versus 73-100% [95-98]. This relatively low reduction success rate in barium enema may be explained by relatively low reduction pressure in the "Rules of Threes" (three attempts of 3 minutes each, with enema bag 3 feet (91 cm) above the fluoroscopy table) [99], to which pediatric radiologists have been strictly adhered.

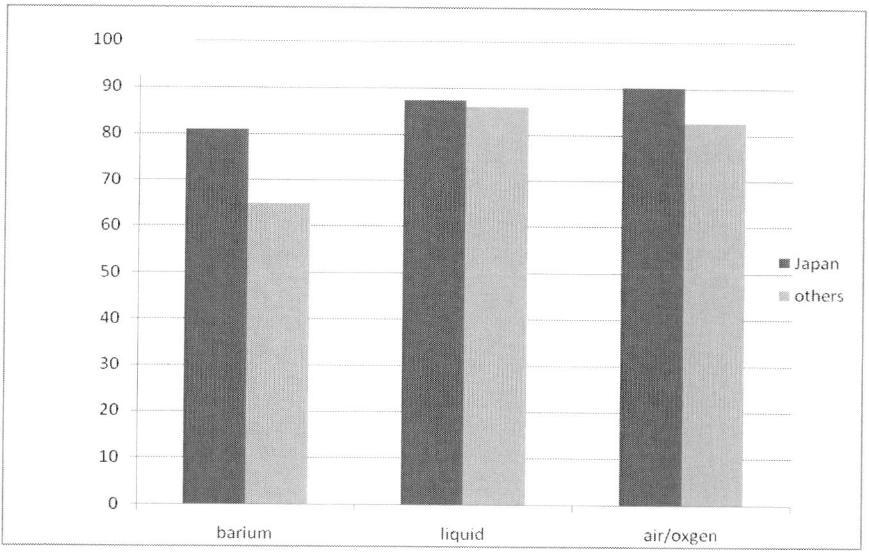

Figure 5. Comparison of reduction success rates of different contrast media in Japan and other countries.

Different from North America and Europe, the health insurance system in Japan allows patients free access to hospitals. The majority of patients with intussusceptions visit clinics or hospitals in a timely fashion and are seen primarily by pediatricians with a surgeon in attendance or by pediatric surgeons. Average reduction success rate of 81.0% (3088/3811) in barium enema under fluoroscopy in Japan [48, 52, 53, 56, 60, 66, 100-104] is much higher than 64.8% (2601/4013) in other countries [9, 14, 16, 30, 57, 61-63, 65, 67, 68, 86, 95, 96, 98, 105-114] (Figure 5). This difference may be due to higher pressure (100~120 cmH_2O) applied in reduction in Japan. On the other hand, average reduction success rates in the Japanese literature was 87.3% (1319/1511) in liquid (water-soluble contrast media) [39, 51, 56, 58, 89, 91, 115-119] enama, and 90.2% (707/784) in air enama [12, 49, 50, 56, 71, 120]. In comparison, average reduction success rates in other countries were, 86.0%

(1579/1836) in liquid enema (normal saline, Hartman's solution, tap water, and water-soluble contrast media) [33, 40, 54, 55, 61, 69, 70, 72, 74, 77, 78, 112, 113, 121] and 82.7% (3496/4226) in air or oxygen enama [10, 29, 36, 38, 41, 46, 47, 64, 73, 75, 76, 86, 95-98, 106, 112, 122-134] (Figure 5). In Japanese institutions, therefore, either Gastrografin® (diluted 1:5 [115]) or air is chosen as a contrast media.

The reduction rates of these two contrast media are comparable, leaving the selection to the clinician's favor.

Recently, Beres, A.L. and Baird, R. [135] reported systematic review with meta-analysis of pneumatic versus hydrostatic reduction, and concluded that pneumatic reduction should be the method of choice. But comparison was made mostly between air reduction and barium reduction in this review. Comparative studies of gas (air and oxygen gas) versus liquid (water-soluble contrast media, normal saline, and Hartman's solution) would be necessary.

Pressure for Enema

Traditional practice in Japan dictates a barium column of 100 cm to a maximum of 120 cm if the intussusception is static [51, 102-104]. Same rule is applied in liquid enema reduction under fluoroscopy [115,118] and sonography [51, 117].

In air enema reduction under fluoroscopy and sonography, air is carefully pumped into the rectum up to a pressure of 80 mmHg at first, which is equivalent to 1-m column of barium [95, 96]. The pressure may be increased to 100 mmHg [49, 71] and to a maximum limit of 120 mmHg [46, 47, 73, 76], which is equivalent approximately to 1.5-m barium column [47]. Guo, J.B. et al. [59] stated that the maximum pressure in young infants should be limited to 80 mmHg. For air reduction, pressure needs to be carefully monitored by pressure gauge [47, 59, 73, 75], which may require a pressure release device and an experienced operator. Once perforation occurs, an emergent tap of the peritoneal cavity by an 18 gauge needle is necessary for tension pneumoperitoneum [46, 47, 84].

Recommendation

25. Liquid enema using diluted Gastrografin® is started with caution at a pressure of 100 cmH_2O and gradually increased to a maximum limit of 120 cmH_2O (equivalent to 94 mmHg). With gas reduction, gas is inflated into the rectum at the initial pressure of 80 mmHg which may

be increased up to 120 mmHg. In infants under 6 months of age who have a higher risk of perforation, the starting pressure of liquid and gas enemas should be 80 cmH_2O and 60 mmHg, respectively, and great attention should be paid to the increase of pressure (recommendation B). Notwithstanding, there is always a risk of perforation.

Current Management in Japan

The pressure limit for 10 months old infant was 120 cmH_20 for liquid reduction in the majority (93%) (Figure 6), and that for 3 months old infant was 100 cmH_20 in the majority (84%) (Figure 7).

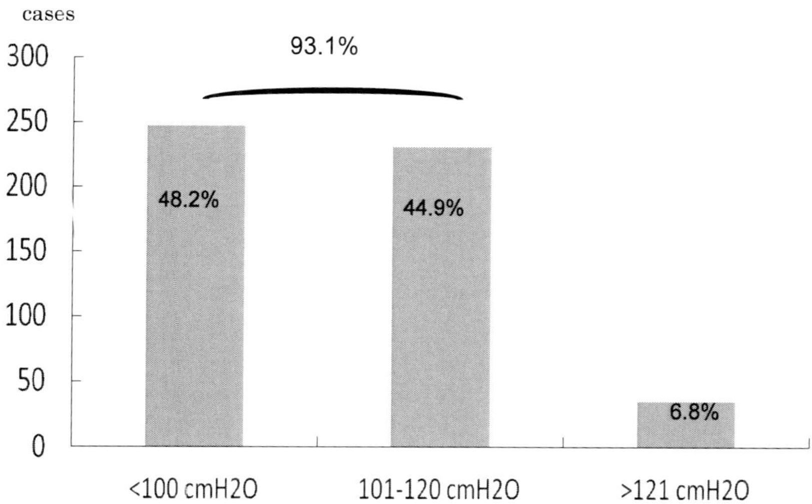

Figure 6. Replies to the question, "If you perform liquid enema what maximum pressure do you apply on a 10 months old infant?" (n = 512).

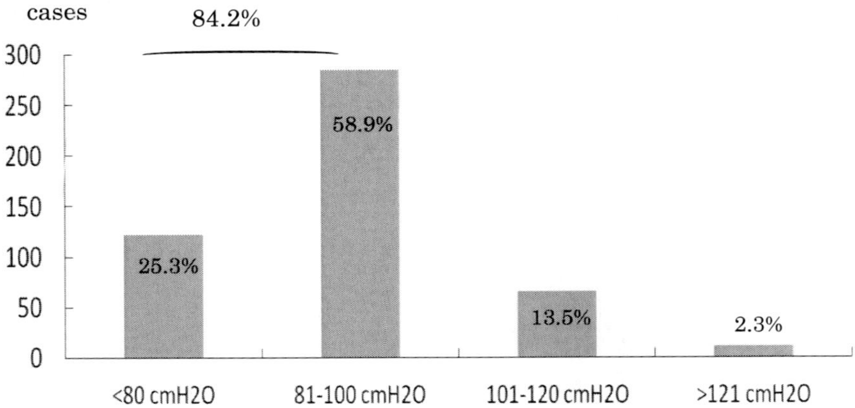

Figure 7. Replies to the question, “If you perform liquid enema what maximum pressure do you apply on a 3 months old infant?” (n = 482).

The pressure limits for 10 months old infant was 120 mmHg for air reduction in the majority (96%) (Figure 8), and that for 3 months old infant was 100 mmHg in the majority (88%) (Figure9).

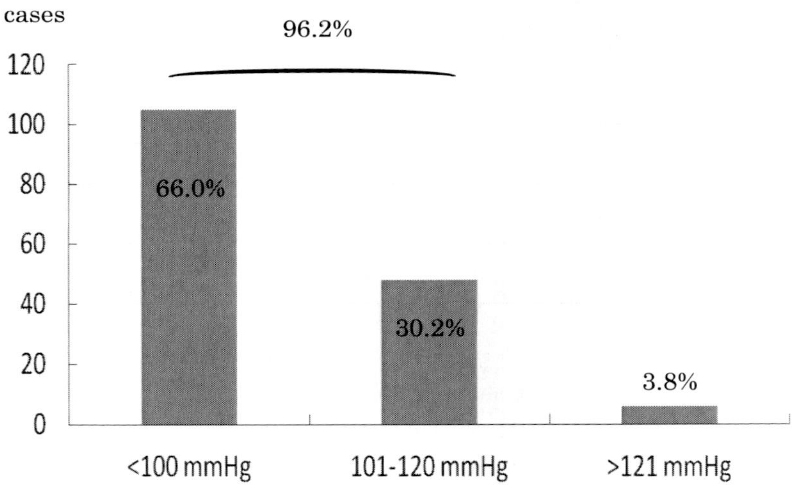

Figure 8. Replies to the question, “If you perform air enema what maximum pressure do you apply on a 10 months old infant?”(n = 159).

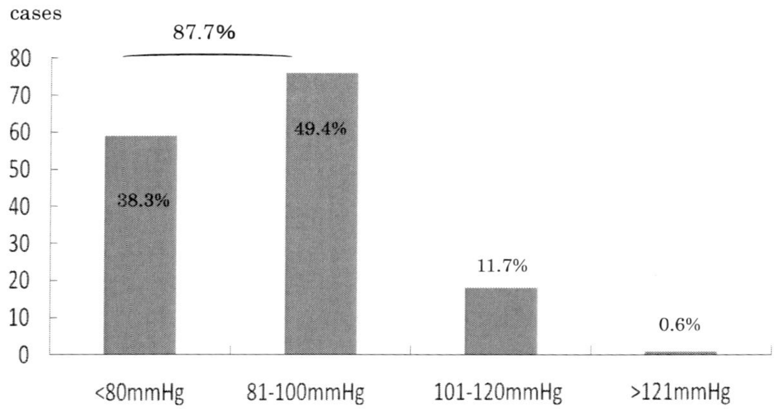

Figure 9. Replies to the question, "If you perform air enema what maximum pressure do you apply on a 3 months old infant?" (n = 154).

Relationship between Maximum Reduction Pressure and Reduction Success Rate

The correlation between maximum reduction pressure and reduction success rate in the different contrast media, including Japanese literatures [2] is illustrated in Figure 10. Reduction success rate correlates well with reduction pressure,

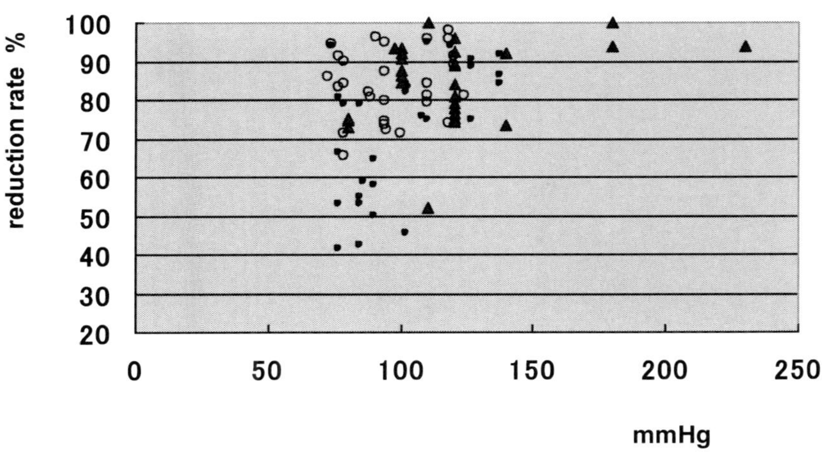

Figure 10. Relationship between maximum reduction pressure and reduction success rate in different contrast media [2] (● Barium, ▲Air, ○Water-soluble contrast).

Complications

The most important potential complication of enema is bowel perforation. There are many reports of high perforation rates by air enema reduction (6.0% [41], 3.9% [76], 2.8% [29]). However, Guo, J.B. et al. [59] reported a very low perforation rate with air enema of 0.141% in 6,396 intussusceptions. Accordingly, the overall mean perforation rate of air enema became extremely low, and perforation rates for air versus liquid enema are reported not to be significantly different in multiple reviews. But Guo's report was excluded from the analysis in the guidelines as the results of critical evaluation [2]. Consequently, perforation rates differed depending on contrast media.

Perforation rates with barium, liquid, and air were 0.14%, 0.37%, and 0.76% respectively [2]. When the perforation rates were confined only in Japanese literatures, they were 0.16% (6/3811) in barium enema [48, 52, 53, 56, 60, 66, 100-104], 0.20% (3/1511) in liquid enema [39, 51, 56, 58, 89, 91, 115-119], and 0.38% (3/784) in air enema [12, 49, 50, 56, 71, 120] (Figure 11). Perforation rate was higher in air than barium or liquid possibly due to the higher pressure applied during pneumatic reduction.

It is clear that the use of excessive pressure during enema reduction is the main cause of perforation [84]. However, perforation does occur at pressures even as low as 60-80 mmHg [84].

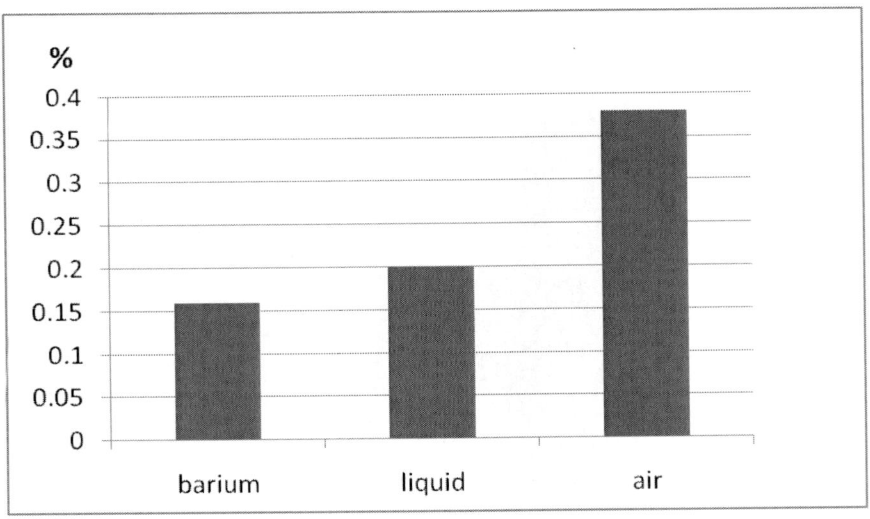

Figure 11. Perforation rates of different contrast media in Japan.

The statistical analysis of perforation shows that more than half of perforations occur in infants less than 6 months of age [2] (Figure 12). Particular care regarding enema reduction should be taken in younger children with a longer duration of symptoms or with evidence of small bowel obstruction on plain radiography [29, 34]. An overly aggressive approach must be condemned in cases with risk factors.

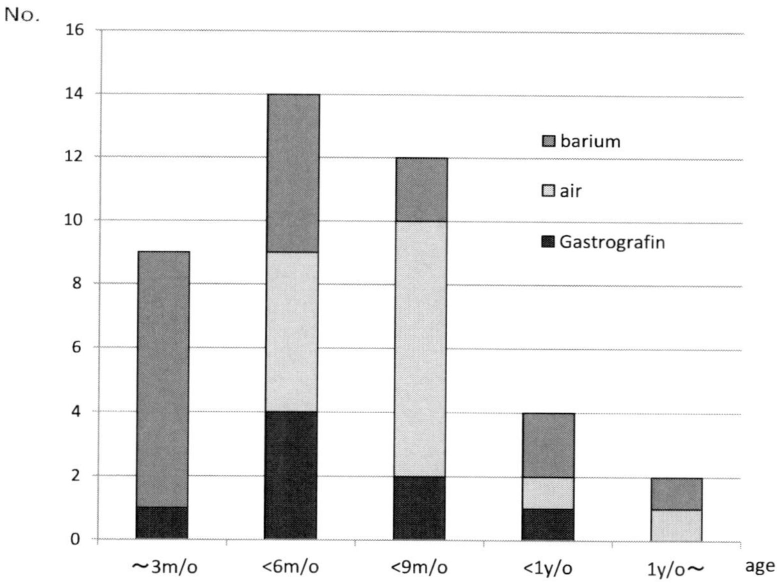

Figure 12. Relationship between age and perforations [2].

Delayed Repeat Enema

Delayed repeat enema refers to reattempt of enema reduction at a certain time interval after the initial attempt at reduction was a failure. It generally refers to reattempt of reduction at the same institution.

Operative reduction is the standard treatment after the failure of enema reduction of intussusceptions. However, 10-14% of intussusceptions have been found to be spontaneously reduced at operation [105, 107]. Hence, enema reduction was repeated at a certain time interval after the first failed attempt. Reduction success rates were improved by 50-86% in DRE cases with failed initial enema reduction [54, 121, 125, 126, 130, 136, 137]. The indications for

DRE are clinically stable infants with no evidence of peritonitis and only when the initial enema achieved a partial reduction [125, 130, 136]. It is believed that partial reduction and the time interval between attempts allow the venous congestion and edema of the bowel wall to decrease and facilitate the reduction of the residual bowel. [54, 125] Optimal timing for the repeat attempt has not been established, but 30 minutes to 4 hours delay after the initial attempt seems to be common [121, 125, 126, 130, 136, 137]. Delayed enema should not be performed if the child is clinically unstable or if the initial enema failed to move the intussusception at all [27, 125, 136].

Recommendation

26. DRE improves reduction success rate. It is useful to attemt DRE, if the initial enema partially reduced the intussusception and if the patient is in stable condition (recommendation B).

Current Management in Japan

DRE (defined as reattempt of reduction at the same institution) was performed mostly after 1 hour (55%, 18 respondents) of those who do DRE (n = 33). DRE was attempted once in 44%, twice in 22%, and 3 times in 33% of respondents who do it with 1 hour intervals (Figure 12).

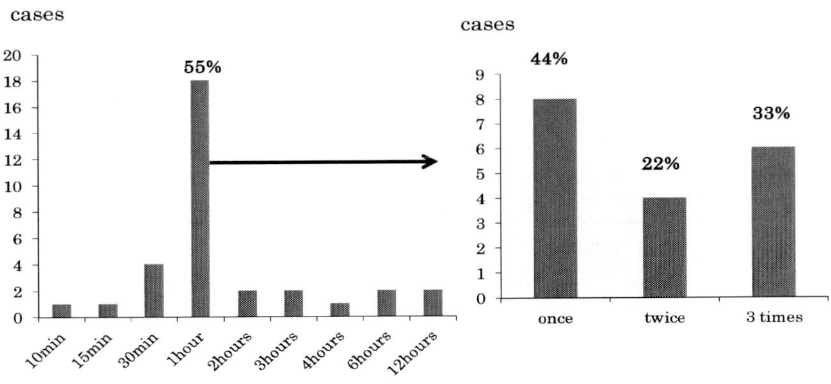

Figure 13. Replies to the questions, "How long is the interval of your delayed repeat enema (n = 33)" and "how many times do you attempt at 1hour interval (n = 18)?"

Admission

Observation under admission is the standard care after a successful enema reduction in Japan. One has to be especially careful in regards to recurrence, because 40% of recurrences take place within 48 hours of the primary reduction of intussusceptions [138]. However, there are several reports in which uncomplicated patients with good hydration, no underlying diseases, and good access to hospitals are able to go home after short-term observation at the outpatient clinic or emergency room [108, 129, 131]. Recurrence of intussusception outside the hospital did not affect clinical outcomes [129].

Recommendation

27. It is allowable to let the patient go home after an appropriate time of observation at an out-patient clinic or emergency room, when the patient is in stable condition and has good access to medical facilities (recommendation C1).

Current Management in Japan

96% (640/669) of respondents replied that they admitted patients almost always for observation after successful reduction.

Antimicrobial Therapy

Serial blood culture studies both pre-enema and post-enema did not justify routine administration of antibiotics after enema reduction [139]. Antibiotics are not routinely used at most institutions [93, 140]. Antimicrobial therapy is justified only in the presence of an underlying sepsis.

Recommendation

28. Routine administration of antimicrobial drugs is not necessary after enema reduction (recommendation C1).

Current Management in Japan

Routine antibiotic cover was denied in 92% (615/667) of respondents.

Confirmation

Reduction is deemed to be satisfactory only if there is free reflux of contrast media into the distal small bowel loops without filling defect under fluoroscopy, together with resolution of symptoms and signs in the patients.

The same thing can be true for air enema [73, 76] or liquid enema [69, 141] under sonography. Sonography is useful to confirm complete reduction repeatedly in uncertain cases without free reflux of contrast media or with persistent filling defect of possible edema, suspected residual bowel or PLP [21, 27, 141]. Edema of the ileocecal valves remains after successful reduction as a post-reduction "donut sign," which is smaller than the target sign and not multi-concentric as is the target sign [27, 142].

Recommendations

29. Sonography is the most effective method to confirm complete reduction and to exclude residual intussusception or recurrence (recommendation B).

Recurrence

In the review of the Japanese literature [2], PLPs were seen in 3.9% (80 PLPs out of 2069 intussusceptions), and the overall recurrence rate of intussusception after enema reduction was an average of 10.3% (392 recurrences out of 3817 intussusceptions) [2].

Daneman, A. et al. [143] found that PLPs were present in 14% of the children who had two or more recurrences compared to 4% of those children who had only one recurrence. More than two recurrences after the initial enema reduction is the predictor of the presence of a PLP.

The age of the patient may be considered a predictor of the presence of PLP, particularly when the intussusception occurs in children older than 4-5 years of age [80, 144], or in recurrent cases in children older than 2 years of age [145]. Lymphoma patients who presented with intussusception ranged in age from 3 to 19 years (median 10 years) [146].

Small intestinal intussusception due to PLP has a high incidence in Peutz-Jehgers syndrome and Henoch-Schonlein purpura. Sonographic findings are of particular value in identifying the rare instances of reduced PLP [80].

Two-thirds of PLPs were identified at ultrasound and 40% of PLPs were diagnosed on barium enema, while air enema had a lower rate of detection of 11% [80]. CT is indicated when sonography fails to identify a suspected PLP [80].

Recommendation

30. In repeated episodes of more than twice or in older children, there is a higher risk of PLPs. Sonography on enema reduction is the most helpful method to detect PLPs (recommendation C1).

Operative Reduction

Operative reduction refers to the Hutchinson procedure by laparotomy in general, but recent laparoscopic reduction is an alternative.

It is important to distinguish between indication and contraindication of enema reduction. Children with evidence of peritonitis, sepsis, or free air on abdominal radiographs are not candidates for enema reduction [27, 147, 148]. These children should be stabilized first and then treated surgically. If a patient is resuscitated from hypovolemic shock and clinically stabilized, enema reduction may be attempted [27, 147, 148]. Operative treatment is also indicated when enema reduction has failed and a PLP was demonstrated or when a PLP is suspected in cases of multiple recurrence [147, 148]. However, multiple recurrences are not a contraindication to attempt enema reduction.

Nonoperative reduction is not expected to be successful in intussusceptions limited to the small bowel.

Indications for bowel resection are perforation of the bowel, necrotic bowel, possibly irreversible ischemia of the bowel, presence of a PLP, and operatively irreducible bowel [147, 148]. Practically, there may be occasions when it is difficult to judge whether the ischemia of the bowel is reversible or not. If there is doubt in regards to the reversibility of the bowel ischemia, it may be safer to resect the bowel and anastomose end-to-end.

Highly mobile cecum has been implicated in the pathogenesis of intussusceptions. Therefore, many surgeons have performed severance of the ileocecal band, suturing the terminal ileum to the ascending colon (ileopexy) or an appendectomy [147, 148] to encourage fixation of the cecum and to prevent future appendicitis. However, these procedures did not necessarily decrease the recurrence rate [148-150].

There is no significant difference in operation time or complications between laparoscopic procedures and open surgery. There are reports of shorter hospital stay and earlier oral intake in the laparoscopic group compared with the open surgery group [151-153]. Disadvantages of laparoscopic procedures include bowel wall injury and difficulty in identification of PLPs [150]. Conversion to open surgery is seen in about 12.5-32% of cases [150-153]. Laparoscopic reduction of intussusception is not covered by health insurance in Japan at present.

Recommendations

31. Operation is indicated in uncorrectable shock, suspect of bowel necrosis/perforation, peritonitis, irreducible intussusceptions, and the presence of PLPs (recommendation A).
32. Bowel resection is indicated in the presence of bowel necrosis /perforation, PLPs, and operatively irreducible intussusceptions (recommendation A).
33. There is no evidence to support additional procedures of ileopexy, severance of ilececal band, or appendectomy to prevent recurrences (recommendation C2).
34. Earlier start of oral intake and shorter hospitalization can be expected following laparoscopic procedures in comparison with open procedures (recommendation C1).

Current Management in Japan

Additional procedures to prevent recurrence and/or future appendicitis were performed almost always in 9.6% (14/146), occasionally in 13.6% (19/146), and never in 77.4% (113/146).

Laparoscopic reduction was selected almost always in 16.9% (25 /148) of respondents, occasionally in 9.5% (14/148), and never in 73.6% (109/148).

Conclusion

These guidelines are aimed to be used specifically in Japan, but some portions may be of value in other countries as well. However, care must be taken to the fact that these guidelines reflect the Japanese medical environment including the health insurance system.

First, the health insurance system in Japan allows patients free access to hospitals without limitation. The majority of patients with intussusceptions are seen primarily by pediatricians with a surgeon in attendance or by pediatric surgeons from the beginning of their treatment. It is very rare that pediatric radiologists join in the team.

Second, medical expenses of infants and children are covered by health insurance and municipal medical aids, and therefore families do not need to pay fees at all in most cases. It is advised that these guidelines should be modified when they are used in other countries to fit their medical environments. In addition, one should judge each individual clinical situation in accordance with staff numbers, experiences, available devices, and the patient's condition.

References

[1] Japanese Society of Emergency Pediatrics. Evidence-based guidelines for the management of intussusception in children. Tokyo, Herusu-shuppan; 2012. (in Japanese)

[2] Ito, Y.; Kusakawa, I.; Murata, Y.; et al. (2012). Japanesse guidelines for the management of intussusceptions in children. 2011. *Pediatrics International;* 54, 948-958, e35-e42.

[3] Ito, Y.; Kusakawa, I.; Murata, Y.; et al. (2012). Management of pediatric intussusceptions in Japan: Results of a postal survey, *Journal of Japanese Society of Emergency Pediatrics,* 11, 396-401. (in Japanese with English abstract)

[4] Ministry of Health, Labour and Welfare. Survey on the effects of introduction of DPC (Diagnosis Procedure Combination) [online]. 2012 [Cited in 2014, August 26] Available from URL: http://www.mhlw.go.jp/bunya/iryouhoken/database/sinryo/dpc.html (in Japanese)

[5] Ministry of Health, Labour and Welfare. Changes in the number of live birth. [online]. 2014 [Cited in 2014, August 28] Available from URL:http://www.mhlw.go.jp/toukei/saikin/hw/jinkou/geppo/nengai13/dl/h3_4.pdf (in Japanese)

[6] Chang, H.G.; Smith, P.F.; Ackelsberg, J.; et al. (2001). Intussusception, Rotavirus Diarrhea, and Rotavirus Vaccine Use Among Children in New York State. *Pediatrics*; 108, 54-60.

[7] Japanese Society of Pathology. Annual of the Pathological Autopsy Cases in Japan. Vol 32-Vol 51, 1990-2009. (in Japanese)

[8] Bruce, J.; Hoo, Y.S.; Cooney, D.R.; et al. (1987). Intussusception: Evolution of current management. *J. Pediatr. Gastroenterol. Nutr.*; 6: 663-764.

[9] Chung, J.L.; Kong, M.S.; Lin, J.N.; et al. (1994). Intussusception in infants and children: Risk factors leading to surgical reduction. J. *Formos. Med. Assoc*; 93: 481-485.

[10] Kaiser, A.D.; Applegate, K.E.; Ladd, A.P. (2007). Current success in the treatment of intussusception on children. *Surgery* ;142: 469-477.

[11] Bines, J.E.; Kohl, K.S.; Forester, J.; et al.(2004). Acute intussusception in infants and children as an adverse event following immunization: case definition and guidelines of data collection, analysis, and presentation. Vaccine; 22, 569-574.

[12] Katsushima, N. (1981). Epidemiology, clinical features and diagnosis of intussusceptions. *Jpn. J. Pediatr. Surg*; 13: 563-570. (in Japanese with English abstract)

[13] Losek, J.D.; Fiete, R.L. (1991). Intussusception and the diagnostic value of testing stool for occult blood. *Am. J. Emerg. Med*; 9, 1-3.

[14] West, K.W.; Stephens, B.; Vane D.W.; et al. (1987) Intussusception: current management in infants and children. Surgery; 102:704-710.

[15] Godbole, A.; Concannon, P.; Glasson, M. (2000). Instructive Case Intussusception presenting as profound lethargy. *J. Paediatr. Child* Health; 36, 392-394.

[16] Reijnen, J,A.; Festen, C.; van Roosmalen, R,P. (1990) Intussusception: factors related to treatment. *Arch. Dis. Child*; 65, 871-873.

[17] Willetts, I,E.; Kite, P.; Barclay, G,R.; et al. (2001). Endotoxin, cytokines and lipid peroxides in children with intussusception. *British Journal of Surgery;* 88, 878-883.

[18] Sargent, M,A.; Babyn, P.; Alton, D.J. (1994). Plain abdominal radiography in suspected intussusception: a reassessment. *Pedatr. Radiol*; 24, 17-20.

[19] Lee, J.M.; Kim, H,; Byun, J.Y.; et al. (1994). Intussusception: characteristic radiolucencies on the abdominal radiograph. *Pedatr. Radiol.*; 24, 293-295.

[20] Daneman, A.; Navarro, O. (2003). Intussusception Part 1: A review of diagnostic approaches. *Pediatr. Radiol.*; 33, 79-85.

[21] Pracros, J.P.; Tran-Minh, V.A.; Morin de Finfe, C.H.; et al. (1987). Acute intestinal intussusception in children. Contribution of ultrasonography (145 cases) *Ann. de Radiol.*; 30:525-530.

[22] Bhisitkul, D.M.; Listernick, R.; Shkolnik, A.; et al. (1992). Clinical application of ultrasonography in the diagnosis of intussusception. *J. Pedatr;* 121, 182-186.

[23] Verschelden, P.; Filiatraut, D.; Garel, L.; et al. (1992). Intussusception in children: Reliability of US in diagnosis –A prospective study. *Radiology*; 184, 741-744.

[24] del-Pozo, G.; Albilos, J.C.; Tejedor, D. (1996). Intussusception: US findings with pathologic correlation –The crescent-in-doughnut sign. *Radioligy;* 199, 688-692.

[25] Teele, R.L.; Vogel, S.A. (1998). Intussusception: the paediatric radiologist's perspective. *Pedatr Surg Int*; 14, 158-162.

[26] Cox, T.D.; Winters, W.D.; Weinberger, E. (1996). CT of intussusceptions in the pediatric patient: diagnosis and pitfalls. *Pediatr Radiol;* 26, 26-32.

[27] Daneman, A.; Navaro, O. (2004). Intussusception Part 2: An update on *the evolution of management*; 34, 97-108.

[28] Applegate, K.E. (2009). Intussusception in children: evidence-based diagnosis and treatment. *Pediatr. Radiol.*; 39, Suppl 2 S140-143.

[29] Stein, M.; Alton, D.J.; Daneman, A. (1992). Pneumatic reduction of intussusception: 5-year experience. *Radiology;* 183, 681-684.

[30] Jennings, C.; Kelleher, J. (1984). Intussusception: influence of age on reducibility. *Pediatr Radiol*;14, 292-294.

[31] Takahashi, T.; Okazaki, T.; Watayo, H.; et al. (2009). Radiolographic signs predictive of success of hydrostatic reduction of intussusception. *Pediatr Surg Int*; 25, 977-980.

[32] Ong, N.T.; Beasley, S.W. (1990). Progression of intussusception. *J. Pediatr Surg* ;25, 644-646.

[33] Peh, W.C.; Khong, P.L.; Lam, C.; et al. (1997). Ileoileocolic intussusception in children: diagnosis and significance. *Br. J. Radiol*; 70, 891-896.

[34] Barr, L.L.; Stansberry.; S.D.; Swischuk, L.E. (1990). Significance of age, duration, obstruction and the dissection sign in intussusception. *Pediatr. Radiol*; 20, 454-456.

[35] Lam, A.H.; Firman, K. (1992). Value of sonography including color Doppler in the diagnosis and management of long standing intussusceptions. *Pediatr. Radiol.*; 22, 112-114.

[36] Lim, H.K.; Bae, S.H.; Lee, K.H.; et al. (1994). Assessment of reducibility of ileocolic intussusception in children: usefulness of color Doppler sonography. *Radiology;* 191, 781-785.

[37] Lagalla, R.; Caruso, G.; Novara, V.; et al. (1994). Color Doppler ultrasonography in pediatric intussusception. *J. Ultrasound. Med.*; 13, 171-174.

[38] Kong, M.S.; Wong, H.F.; Lin, S.L.; et al. (1997). Factors related to detection of blood flow by color Doppler ultrasonography in intussusception. *J. Ultrasound. Med.*; 16, 141-144.

[39] Yoshida, F.; Kamagata, S.; Hirobe, S.; et al. (2007). Treatment of intussusceptions in children – Do guidelines for treatment change with the use of a Power Doppler? – *J. Abdom. Emerg. Med.*; 27, 721-724. (in Japanese with English absract)

[40] del-Pozo, G.; Gonzalez-Spinola, J.; Gomez-Anson, B.; et al. (1996). Intussusception: trapped peritoneal fluid detected with US--relationship to reducibility and ischemia. *Radiology*; 201, 379-83.

[41] Britton, I.; Wilkinson, AG. (1999). Ultrasound features of intussusception predicting outcome of air enema. *Pediatr. Radiol.*; 29, 705-710.

[42] Shanbhogue, R.L.; Hussain, S.M.; Meradji. M.; et al. (1994). Ultrasonography is accurate enough for the diagnosis of intussusception. *J. Pediatr. Surg.;* 29, 324-328.

[43] Jen, H.C.; Shew, S.B. (2009). The impact of hospital type and experience on the operative utilization in pediatric intussusception: a nationwide study. *J. Pediatr. Surg.*; 44, 241-246.

[44] Bratton, S.L.; Haberkern, C.M.; Waldhausen, J.H.T.; et al. (2001). Intussusception: Hospital size and risk of surgery. *Pediatrics*; 107, 299-303.

[45] Somme, S.; To, T.; Langer, J.C. (2006). Factors determining the need for operative reduction in children with intussusception: a population-based analysis. *J Pediatr Surg*; 41, 1014-1019.

[46] Katz, M.; Phelan, E.; Carlin, J.B.; et al. (1993). Gas enema for the reduction of intussusception: relationship between clinical signs and symptoms and outcome. *Am. J. Roentgenol.*; 160, 363-366.
[47] Gu, L.; Alton, D.J.; Daneman, A.; et al. (1988). Intussusception reduction in children by rectal insufflation of air. *AJR Am. J. Roentgenol;* 150, 1345-8.
[48] Minam,i A.; Fujii, K.; et al. (1975). Intussusception in children: hydrostatic reduction. *Am. J. Dis. Child*; 129, 346-348.
[49] Kitamura, T. (1981). The pneumatic reduction for patients with intussusceptions during infancy and childhood. *Jpn. J. Pediatr. Surg*; 13, 621-626. (Japanese with English absract)
[50] Tamanaha, K.; Wimbish, K.; Talwalkar, Y.B.; et al. (1987). Air reduction of intussusception in infants and children.*J. Pediatr*; 111, 733-736.
[51] Hamabata, H.; Kayo, M.; Nakamura, T.; et al. (1999). Ultrasound-guided hydrostatic reduction of childhood intussusceptions. *Jpn J Pediatr Surg*; 31, 479-483. (in Japanese with English absract)
[52] Suzuk,i M.; Hayakawa, K.; Nishimura, K.; et al. (1999). Intussusception: the role of general anesthesia during hydrostatic barium reduction. *Radiat Med;* 17, 121-124.
[53] Kajimoto, T.; Nozaki, S.; Yoshida, Y. (1981). Hydrostatic pressure reduction by barium enema for intussusception in children. *Jpn. J. Pediatr. Surg*; 13, 613-619. (in Japanese with English absract)
[54] Collins, D.L.; Pinckney, L.E.; Miller, K.E.; et al. (1989). Hydrostatic reduction of ileocolic intussusception: a second attempt in the operating room with general anesthesia. *J. Pediatr*; 115, 204-207.
[55] Roheschneider, W.K.; Troger, J. (1995). Hydrostatic reduction of intussusceptions under US guidance. *Pediatr. Radiol.*; 25, 530-534.
[56] Nagasaki, A.; Zaizen, Y.; Shono, K. (2007). Enema reduction of intussusceptions: 10 years' experience. *J. Abdom Emerg. Med.*; 27, 693-697. (in Japanese with English absract)
[57] Liu, K.W.; MacCarthy, J.; Guiney, E.J.; et al. (1986). Intussusception - current trends in management. *Arch. Dis. Child*; 61, 75-77.
[58] Kotani, T. Banno, K.; Kawakami, N.; et al. (2005). Analysis of 101 cases of intussusception. J Jpn Pediatr Soc; 109, 1027-1030. (in Japanese with English absract)
[59] Ishihara, M.; Azuma, Y.; Okabe, I.; et al. (1984) The effect of glucagon for the barium enema reduction of intussusception. *Jpn J Pediatr Surg*; 16, 107-111. (in Japanese with English abstract)

[60] Guo, J.B.; Ma, X.; Zhou, Q. (1986). Result of air pressure enema of intussusceptions: 6,396 cases in 13 years. *J. Pediatr. Surg*; 12, 1201-1203.

[61] Chan, K.L.; Saing, H.; Peh, W.C.; et al. (1997). Childhood intussusception: ultrasound-guided Hartmann's solution hydrostatic reduction or barium enema reduction? *J. Pediatr. Surg.*; 32, 3-6.

[62] Touloukian, R.J.; O'Connell, J.B.; Markowitz, R.I.; et al. (1987). Analgesic premedication in the management of ileocolic intussusceptions. *Pediatrics*; 79, 432-434.

[63] Hoy, G.R.; Dunbar, D.; Boles, T. (1977). The use of glucagon in the diagnosis and management of ileocolic intussusceptions. *J. Pediatr. Surg.*; 12, 939-944.

[64] McDermott, V.G.; Taylor, T.; Mackenzie, S.; et al. (1994). Pneumatic reduction of intussusception: clinical experience and factors affecting outcome. *Clin. Radiol.*; 49, 30-4.

[65] Paes, R.A.; Hyde, I.; Griffiths, D.M. (1988). The management of intussusceptions. *Br. J. Radiol.*; 61, 187-189.

[66] Oka, Y.; Hayashi, A.; Kamagata, S.; et al. (1999). Barium enema and reduction of intussusception: especially on hydrostatic pressure and it's practice. *Jpn. J. Pediatr. Surg.*; 31, 484-489. (in Japanese with English absract)

[67] Franken, E.A. Jr.; Smith, W.L.; Chernish, S.M.; et al. (1983). The use of glucagon in hydrostatic reduction of intussusception: a double-blind study of 30 patients. *Radiology*; 146, 687-689.

[68] Mortensson, W.; Eklof, O.; Laurin, S. (1984). Hydrostatic reduction of childhood intussusception. The role of adjuvant glucagon medication. *Acta. Radiol. Diagn.*; 25, 261-264.

[69] Woo, S.K.; Kim, J.S.; Suh, S.J.; et al. (1992). Childhood intussusception: US-guided hydrostatic reduction. *Radiology*; 182, 77-80.

[70] Riebel, T.W.; Nasir, R.; Weber, K.; et al. (1993). US-guided hydrostatic reduction of intussusception in children. *Radiology;* 188, 513-516.

[71] Todani, T.; Sato, Y.; Watanabe, Y.; et al. (1990). Air reduction for intussusception in infancy and childhood: ultrasonographic diagnosis and management without X-ray exposure. Z Kinderchir; 45, 222-226.

[72] Chiu, C.Y.; Tok, T.S. (1993). Intussusception reduction by hydrostatic saline enema under sonographical guidance: clinical experience in 33 cases. *J. Formos. Med. Assoc*; 92, 50-54.

[73] Wang, G.; Liu, X.G.; Zitsman J.L. (1995). Nonfluoroscopic reduction of intussusception by air enema. *World J. Surg.*; 19:435-438.
[74] Choi S.O.; Park W.H.; Woo, S.K.; et al. (1994) Ultrasound-guided water enema: an alternative method of nonoperative treatment for childhood intussusceptions. *J. Pediatr. Surg.*; 29, 498-500.
[75] Gu, L.; Zhu, H.; Wang, S.; et al. (2000). Sonographic guidance of air enema for intussusception reduction in children. *Pediatr. Radiol.*; 30, 339-342.
[76] Yoon, C.H.; Kim, H.J.; Goo, H.W. (2001). Intussusception in children: US-guided pneumatic reduction--initial experience. *Radiology;* 218, 85-88.
[77] Wang, G.; Liu, S. (1988) Enema reduction of intussusceptions by hydrostatic pressure under ultrasound guidance. *J. Pediatr. Surg*; 23, 814-818.
[78] Crystal, P.; Hertzanu, Y.; Farber, B.; et al. (2002). Sonographically guided hydrostatic reduction of intussusception in children. *J. Clin. Ultrasound;* 30, 343-8.
[79] Bolia, A.A. (1985). Case report: Diagnosis and Hydrostatic Reduction of an Intussuception under Ultrasound guidance. *Clin. Radiol.*; 36, 655-657.
[80] Navarro, O.; Dugougeat, F.; Kornecki, A.; et a. (2000). The impact of imaging in the management of intussusception owing to pathologic lead points in children. A review of 43 cases. *Pediatr. Radiol.*; 30, 594–603.
[81] del-Pozo, G.; Albillos, J.C.; Tejedor, D.; et al. (1999). Intussusception in children: current concepts in diagnosis and enema reduction. *Radiographics;* 19, 299-319.
[82] Ravitch, M.M. (1948). Reduction of intussusception by barium enema. *Ann. Surg.*; 128, 904-917.
[83] Ein, S.H.; Mercer, S.; Humphry, A.; et al. (1981). Colon perforation during attempted barium enema reduction of intussusceptions. *J. Pediatr.* Surg.; 16, 313-315.
[84] Daneman, A.; Alton, D.J.; Ein, S.; et al. (1995). Perforation during attempter intussusception reduction in children- a comparison of perforation with barium and air: *Pediatric Radiology*; 19, 81-88.
[85] Nagashima, K.; Tsuchiya, H.; Ohashi, S.; et al. (1999). Four cases of barium peritonitis following hydrostatic reduction. *Jpn. J. Pediatr. Surg.*; 31, 547-551. (in Japanese with English absract)
[86] Palder, S.B.; Ein, S.H.; Stringer, D.A.; et al. (1991). Intussusception: barium or air? *J. Pediatr. Surg*; 26, 271-275.

[87] Sisel, R.J.; Donovan, A.J.; Yellian, A.E. (1972). Experimental fecal peritonitis: Influence of barium sulfate or watersoluble radiographic contrast material on survival. *Arch. Surg.*; 104, 765-768.
[88] Daneman, A.; Alton, D.J. (1996). Intussusception. Issues and controversies related to diagnosis and reduction. *Radiol. Clin. North* Am; 34, 743-756.
[89] Hirama, T.; Nui, A.; Meguro, M.; et al. (1999). Intussusception (organic disorder, recurrence). *Jpn. J. Pediatr. Surg.*; 31, 489-492. (in Japanese with English abstract)
[90] Campbell, J, (1989). Contrast media in intussusceptions. *Pediatr. Radiol.;* 19, 293-296.
[91] Obana, K.; Ogawa, T.; Okinaga, K.; et al. (1999). Gastrografin enema reduction for intussusceptions in infants. *Jpn. J. Pediatr. Surg*; 31, 463-466. (in Japanese with English absract).
[92] Katz, M.E.; Kolm, P. (1992). Intussusception reduction 1991: an international survey of pediatric radiologists. *Pediatr. Radiol.*; 22, 318-322.
[93] Jewell, F.M.; Roobottom, C.; Duncan, A. (1995). Variations in the radiological management of intussusception: results of a postal survey. *British J. Radiol.;* 68, 13-18.
[94] Rosenfeld, K.; McHugh, K. (1999). Survey of intussusception reduction in England, Scotland and Wales: How and why we could do better. *Clinical Radiology;* 54, 452-458.
[95] Phelan, E.; de Campo, J.F.; Malecky, G. (1988). Comparison of oxygen and barium reduction of ileocolic intussusceptions. *Am. J. Roentgenol*; 150, 1349-1352.
[96] Beasley, S.W.; Glover, J. (1992). Intussusception: prediction of outcome of gas enema. *J. Pediatr. Surg.*; 27, 474-475.
[97] Meyer, J.S. (1993). Air and liquid contrast agents in the management of intussusception: controlled, randomized trial. *Radiology;* 188, 507-511..98. 98. 98. Rubi, I.; Vera, R.; Rubi, S.C.; et al. (2002). Air reduction of intussusceptions. *Eur. J. Pediatr. Surg.*; 12, 387-390.
[98] Ravitch, M.M.; McCune, R.M. (1950). Intussusception in infancy and children. *J. Pediatr*; 37, 153-173.
[99] Mimatsu, K.; Oida, T.; Nishio, S.; et al. (1998). Clinical study of intussusceptions in infants – analysis of 713 cases. J Jpn Soc Pediatr Surg; 34, 1023-1028. (in Japanese with English absract)

[100] Ohtsu, K.; Furuta, Y.; Ogura, Y. (1999). Hydrostatic pressure reduction by barium enema for intussusceptions in children. *Jpn. J. Pediatr. Surg.*; 31, 459-462. (in Japanese with English absract)
[101] Okuyama, H.; Nakai, H.; Okada, A. (1999). Is barium enema reduction safe and effective in patients with a long duration of intussusception? *Pediatr. Surg. Int.*; 15, 105-7.
[102] Imaizumi, S.; Iwanaka, T.; Arai, M.; et al. (2000). Intussusception in children – a 17-year review. *J. Abdom. Emerg. Med.*; 20, 1117-1123. (in Japanese with English absract)
[103] Saito, T.; Yamada, S.; Sato, Y.; Yoshida, H.; et al. (2007). Clinical analyses of 877 children with intussusceptions ata a single center. *Jpn. J. Pediatr. Surg.;* 39, 505-509. (in Japanese with English absract)
[104] Ein, S.H.; Alton, D.; Palder, S.B.; et al. (1997). Intussusception in 1990s: has 25 years made a difference? *Pediatr Surg Int;* 12, 374-376.
[105] Eshel, G.; Barr, J.; Heyman, E. et al. (1997). Intussusception: A 9-year survey (1986-1995). *J. Pediatric Gastroenterology and Nutrition*; 24, 253-256.
[106] Ekloef, O.A.; Johanson, L.; Loehr, G. (1980). Childhood intussusception: hydrostatic reducibility and incience of leading poins in different age groups. *Pediatr Radiol*; 10, 83-86.
[107] Bonadio, W.A. (1988). Intussuscption reduced by barium enema. Outcome and short-term follow-up *Clin. Pediatr*; 27, 601-604.
[108] Bettenay, F.; Beasley, S.W.; de Campo, J.F.; et al. (1988). Intussusception: clinical prediction of outcome of barium reduction. *Aust. N. Z. J. Surg.;* 58, 899-902.
[109] Skipper, R.P.; Boeckman, C.R.; Klein, R.L. (1990). Childhood intussusception. *Surg. Gynecol. Obstet*; 171 151-3.
[110] Le Masne, A.; Lortat-Jacob, S.; Sayegh, N.; et al. (1999). Intussusception in infants and children: feasibility of ambulatory management. *Eur. J. Pediatr*; 158, 707-10.
[111] Hadidi, A.T.; El Shal, N. (1999). Childhood intussusception: A comparative study of nonsurgical management. *J. Pediatr. Surg.*; 34, 304-307
[112] Shehata, S.; El Kholi, N.; Sultan, A.; et al. (2000). Hydrostatic reduction of intussusception: barium, air, or saline? Pediatr Surg Int; 16, 380-2.
[113] Koumanidou, C.; Vakaki, M.; Pitsoulakis, G.; et al. (2002) Sonographic detection of lymph nodes in the intussusception of infants and young children: clinical evaluation and hydrostatic reduction. *AJR Am. J. Roentgenol.*; 178, 445-50.

[114] Okazaki, T.; Ogasawara. Y.; Nakazawa, N.; et al. (2006). Reduction of intussusception in infants by pediatric surgical team:improvement in safety and outcome. *Pediatr Surg. Int.*; 22, 897-900.

[115] Hoshino, M.; Asai, Y.; Inoue, M.; et al. (2007). Intussusception observed in infancy and children. *J. Jpn. Soc. Pediatr. Surg.*; 43, 23-31. (in Japanese with English absract)

[116] Yamashita, M.; Nishijima, E.; Muraji, T.; et al. (2007). A treatment strategy for intussusception. *J. Abdom. Emerg. Med.*; 27, 711-713. (in Japanese with English absract)

[117] Hisamatsu, C.; Yamamoto, T.; Hatakeyama, T et al. (2007). A comparative study of the first hydrostatic pressure for the reduction of intussusceptions. *Jpn J Pediatr Surg*; 39, 510-513. (in Japanese with English absract)

[118] Gotoh, C.; Kitano, Y.; Uchida, H.; et al. (2007). Hydrostatic reduction of Intussusception: A review of 645 cases. *J. Abdom. Emerg. Med.*; 27, 687-692. (in Japanese with English absract)

[119] Suganuma, Y.; Kitamura, T. Satoh, Y.; et al. (1992). Study of air reduction in 119 cases of intussusception - With reference to air pressure and perforation during reduction - . *J. Jpn. Soc. Pediatr. Surg.*; 28, 327-335. (in Japanese with English absract)

[120] Gonzalez-Spinola, J.; Del Pozo, G.; Tejedor, D.; et al. (1999). Intussuseption: the accuracy of ultrasound-guided saline enema and the usefulness of a delayed attempt at reduction. *J. Pediatr. Surg.*; 34, 1016-1020.

[121] Ein, S.H.; Palder, S.B.; Alton, D.J.; et al. (1994). Intussusception: toward less surgery? *J. Pediatr. Surg.*; 29, 433-5.

[122] de Campo, J.F.; Phelan, E. (1989). Gas reduction of intussusception. *Pediatr. Radiol.;* 19, 297-8.

[123] Menor, F.; Cortina, H.; Marco, A. et al. (1992). Effectiveness of pneumatic reduction of ileocolic intussusception in children. *Gastrointest Radiol.*; 17, 339-43.

[124] Saxton, V.; Katz, M.; Phelan, E.; et al. (1994). Intussusception: a repeat delayed gas enema increases the nonoperative reduction rate. *J. Pdiatr. Surg; 29*, 588-589.

[125] Gorenstein, A.; Raucher, A,; Serour, F.; et al. (1998). Intussusception in children: reduction with repeated, delayed air enema. *Radiology*; 206, 721-724.

[126] Heenan, S.D.; Kyriou ,J.; Fitzgerald, M.; et al. (2000). Effective dose at pneumatic reduction of paediatric intussusception. *Clin. Radiol.*, 55, 811-6.
[127] Lui, K.W.; Wong, H.F.; Cheung, Y.C.; et al. (2001). Air enema for diagnosis and reduction of intussusception in children: clinical experience and fluoroscopy time correlation. *J. Pediatr. Surg.*; 36, 479-81.
[128] Bajaj L.; Roback M.G. (2003). Postreduction management of intussusception in a children's hospital emergency department. *Pediatrics;* 112:1302-1307.
[129] Navarro, O.M.; Daneman, A.; Chae, A. (2004). Intussusception: the use of delayed, repeated reduction attempts and the management of intussusceptions due to pathologic lead points in pediatric patients. *AJR;* 182, 1169-1176.
[130] Al-Jazaeri, A.; Yazbeck, S.; Fillatrault, D.; et al. (2006). Utility of hospital admission after successful enema reduction of ileocolic intussusception. *J. Pediatr. Surg.*; 41, 1010-1013.
[131] Shapkina, A.N.; Shapkin, V.V.; Nelubov, I.V.; et al. (2006). Intussusception in children: 11-year experience in Vladivostok. *Pediatr Surg Int;* 22, 901-4.
[132] Cheung, S.T.; Lee, K.H.; Yeung, T.H.; et al. (2007). Minimally invasive approach in the management of childhood intussusception. *ANZ J. Surg;* 77, 778-81.
[133] Ramachndran, P.; Gupta, A.; Vincent, P.; et al. (2008). Air enema for intussusception: Is predicting the outcome important? *Pediatr. Surg. Int*; 24, 311-313.
[134] Beres, A.L.; Baird, R. (2013) An institutional analysis and systematic review with meta-analysis of pneumatic versus hydrostatic reduction for pediatric intussusception. *Surgery;*154:328-334.
[135] Sandler, A.D.; Ein, S.H.; Conolly, B.; et al. (1999). Unsuccessful air-enema reduccton of intussusception: is a second attempt worthwhile? *Pediatr. Surg. Int;* 15, 214-216.
[136] Yoshida, F.; Kamagata, S.; Hirobe, S.; et al. (2007). The Usefulness of delayed repeated enema in intussusception. J Jap Soc Emergency Pediatrics;6:200-204. (in Japanese with English absract)
[137] Ekloef, O.; Reiter, S. (1978). Recurrent intussusception. Analysis of a series treated with hydrostatic reduction. *Acta Radiolo Diagn*;19, 250-258.

[138] Somekh, E.; Serour, F.; Goncalves, P.; et al. (1996). Air enema for reduction of intussusception in children: risk of bacteremia. *Radiology;* 200, 217-218.

[139] Meyer, J.S. (1992). The current radiologic management of intussusception: a survey and review. *Pediatr. Radiol.*; 22, 323-325.

[140] Peh, W.C.G.; Khong, P.L.; Lam, C.; et al. (1999). Reduction of intussusception in children using sonograpic guidance. *AJR;* 173, 985-988.

[141] Rohrschneider, W.; Troeger, J.; Betsch, B. (1994). The postreduction donut sign. *Pediatr. Radiol;* 24, 156-160.

[142] Daneman, A.; Alton, D.J.; Lobo, E.; et al. (1998). Patterns of recurrence of intussusception in children: a 17-year review. *Pediatr. Radiol* 1998; 28: 913-919.

[143] Ong, N.T.; Beasley, S.W. (1990). The leadpoint in intususception. *J. Pediatr Surg;* 25, 640-643.

[144] Beasley, S.W.; Auldist, A.W.; Stokes, K.B. (1987). Recurrent intussusception: barium or surgery? *Aust. N. Z. J. Surg.*; 57, 11-14.

[145] Gupta, H.; Davidoff, A.M.; Pui, C.H.; et al. (2007). Clinical implications and surgical management of intussusceptions in pediatric patients with Burkitt lymphoma. *J. Pediatr. Surg*; 42:998-1001.

[146] Bruce, J.; Huh, Y.S.; Cooney,D.R.; et al. (1987). Intussusception: evolution of current management. *J. Pediatr Gastroenterol Nutr*; 6, 663-674.

[147] Stringer, M.D.; Pablot, S.M.; Brereton, F.J. (1992). Pediatric intussusception. *Br. J. Surg*; 79, 867-876.

[148] Koh, L.C.; Sheu, J.C.; Wang, N.L.; et al. (2006). Recurrent ileocolic intussusception after different surgical procedures in children. *Pediatr Surg. Int.*; 22, 725-728.

[149] Bonnard, A.; Demarche, M.; Dimitriu, C.; et al. (2008). Indications for laparoscopy in the management of intussusception: A multicenter retrospective study conducted by the French Study Group for Pediatric Laparoscopy(GECI). *J. Pediatr. Surg.;* 43, 1249-1253.

[150] Sato, M.; Hamada, Y.; Tanano, A.; et al.(2001). Role of laparoscopic surgery in the treatment of intussusceptions. *J. Jpn. Surg. Assoc.*; 37, 47-51 (Japanese with English absract).

[151] Kia, K.F.; Mony, V.K.; Drongowski, R.A.; et al. (2005). Laparoscopic vs open approach for intussusception requiring operative intervention. *J. Pediatr. Surg.*; 40, 281-284.

[152] Bailey, K.A.; Wales, P.W.; Gerstle, J.T. (2007). Laparoscopic versus open reduction of intussusception in cildren: a single-institution comparative experience. *J. Pediatr. Surg.*; 42, 845-848.

In: Intussusception and Bowel Obstruction ISBN: 978-1-63482-703-4
Editor: Rosie Miller

Chapter 4

Prenatal Intussusception: What Consequences?

***Taieb Chouikh*[1,3]*, Chaima Mrad*[1]*, Awatef Charieg*[1,3]*, Sofiene Ghorbel*[1,3] *and Sonia Benkhalifa*[2,3]**

[1]Department of Pediatric Surgery B Children Hospital of Tunis, Tunisia
[2.]Department of Anesthesiology Children Hospital of Tunis, Tunisia
[3]Tunis School of medicine, El Manar Tunis University, Tunisia

Abstract

Intrauterine bowel intussusception is rare. Foetal intussusception can be responsible of intestinal gangrene and resorption of the intussuscepted portions of the bowel and intestinal atresia may result. Prenatal diagnosis is possible but difficult, the prenatal features remain unknown in 60% of the cases

Postnatally, the newborn presents an acute neonatal occlusion with bilious vomiting and distended abdomen. The diagnosis is currently made during surgery for acute bowel obstruction.

There are few cases described that demonstrate the intrauterine intussusception as a cause of intestinal atresia. When intestinal atresia is discovered an attentive examination of the distal part of the atresia would assist the classification of atresia and help in the understanding of the mechanism of occurrence, and to determine if there is or not an antenatal intussusceptions.

Introduction

Intussusception is rare in the neonatal period. Of about 6000 published cases in the pediatric population, only 28 occurred in the neonatal period [1]. The commonest site was the ileum. The jejunum is an uncommon location. The cause of the intussusception is unknown in majority of the cases. Cases of ileal atresia consequent to intrauterine intusussception have been reported before. Intrauterine intussusceptions causing jejunal atresia is further rare with only few cases described in the literature [2, 3].

It has been suspected that intestinal atresia may be secondary to prolonged bowel ischemia in utero [4], thus a careful examination of distal blind end is important in making the diagnosis.

The most accepted theory to explain intestinal atresia is the vascular incident caused by disorder of mesenteric flow [5] inducing prolonged bowel ischemia in utero. Laufman [6] demonstrated in 1949 that when isolated sterile devascularized loops of intestine were left in the peritoneal cavity, they converted to fibrous bands or disappeared entirely.

The Ischemia can occur prenatally because of intussusception. The incidence of this latter cause of intestinal atresia has been described between 0.6% and 13% [7] or 25% of all ileal atresia [8].

A review of published cases of intrauterine intussusceptions inducing intestinal atresia, reported a total of 80 patients in 31 different publications of intrauterine intussusceptions (between 1975 [9] and 2014 [10] (Table 1), the largest one reported a total of 24 cases [9], in 4 cases [11, 12, 13] a Meckel diverticulum was reported, in one case an associated intestinal duplication was found [12].

We excluded the cases where a volvulus was associated, since we thought that fetal intestinal volvulus may be complicated by ischemia and can lead to intestinal atresia; thus the occurred intussusceptions are not the primary cause for the intestinal atresia.

The sonographic findings of fetal intestinal intussusceptions at term may include a "target-like" lesion; Shimotake [14] reported that this was a round hyperechoic area of fetal bowel surrounded by hypoechoic ring of bowel wall. In other cases the sonographic findings were unspecific and lead to a diagnosis of intestinal obstruction. Intestinal dilation, fetal ascites, meconium pseudocyst or intra-abdominal calcifications have been reported [14].

Ming Kwang Shyu [15], has correlated prenatal ultrasound findings with postnatal outcome and defined persistent ascites, pseudocyst or dilated bowel loops as highly predictive of need for postnatal surgery (92%). Therefore, once diagnosed, pregnant women with fetal anomalies should deliver in a tertiary care centre where immediate neonatal and pediatric surgical facilities are available.

An abnormal prenatal ultrasound finding was reported in 11% of the reported cases. The prenatal features remain unknown in 60% of the cases.

Intrauterine Intussusception causing Intestinal Atresia is usually seen in full-term neonates but has been reported rarely in prematurely born neonates.

The condition is considered to occur very late in pregnancy, which is supported by presence of normal or near-normal sized colon due to passage of meconium in majority of these neonates and absence of associated anomalies [8, 9, 16].

In the intestinal atresias owing to intussusceptions in which a barium enema was carried out, a normal or nearly normal-sized colon was revealed, in contrast to other types of low intestinal obstruction, which are described as microcolon or unused colon. This suggests that intrauterine intussusception could occur during the last phases of gestation.

After Birth, in 29% of the reported cases, the newborn presents an acute neonatal occlusion with bilious vomiting abdominal distension. Abdominal radiography is sufficient to indicate surgery, and intestinal opacification is rarely needed.

Surgical management includes a small bowel resection and end-to-end anastomosis or a primary intestinal derivation with a delayed anastomosis. The prognosis of this entity is good, and follow up in most of the time is uneventful.

In 14% of the antenatal intussusceptions reported cases the ileal atresia was Type 2, according to the classification of Grosfeld [17], while Type 3, where a mesenteric gap due to a mesenteric thrombosis, was reported in 18% of the cases. The type of the atresia remains unclear in 68% of the cases.

- *Type I* is represented by a transluminal membrane or short atretic segment causing complete intestinal bowel obstruction
- *Type II* has the blind ending proximal bowel attached to the collapsed and undelveloped distal bowel by a fibrous cord along the edge of mesentery. There is no mesenteric defect.
- *Type III* is similar to type II except that the fibrous connecting cord is absent and there is a V-shaped meseneteric defect, such as 3 cases of our study.
- *Type IV* represents multiple segment atresias like a string of sausages or a combination of types I and III

Table 1. Summary of published cases on Intrauterine Intussusception

Study Number	Authors	Year of publication	Reported cases	Antenatal Diagnosis	Type atresia
1	Todani T and et al. (9)	1975	24	Unknown	Unknown
2	Aubert D and et al. (21)	1982	1	Unknown	Unknown
3	Pavri DR and et al. (22)	1983	1	Unknown	Unknown
4	Hayashida Y and et al. (19)	1984	4	Unknown	Unknown
5	Reed DN Jr and et al. (3)	1987	1	No	3A
6	Woodall DL and et al. (23)	1987	1	Unknown	Unknown
7	Brinson RA and et al. (24)	1988	1	Unknown	Unknown
8	Adejuyigbe O and et al. (25)	1990	1	No	3A
9	Akgür F and et al. (26)	1991	1	Unknown	Unknown
10	Kelly SB and et al. (27)	1991	1	No	Unknown
11	Das PC and et al. (28)	1992	1	Unknown	Unknown
12	Zijlmans CW and et al. (29)	1993	1	Unknown	Unknown
13	De Luca U and et al. (7)	1995	1	Yes	2
14	Gündoğdu HZ and et al. (30)	1996	2	No	Unknown
15	Réguerre Y and al(12)	1997	2	Yes 1case No 1 case	Unknown
16	Imai Y and al(18)	1999	11	Yes 1 case	3A: 8 cases 2 : 3 cases
17	Shimotake T and et al. (14)	2000	1	Yes	3A
18	MachmouchiM and et al. (31)	2000	1	No	Unknown
19	Rattan KN and et al. (20)	2000	1	No	Unknown
20	Mcheik JN and et al. (32)	2003	1	No	2

Study Number	Authors	Year of publication	Reported cases	Antenatal Diagnosis	Type atresia
21	Kilic N and et al. (13)	2003	1	Unknown	Unknown
22	Yang JI and et al. (33)	2004	2	Yes	Unknown
23	Komuro H and et al. (8)	2004	11	Unknown	2
24	Huang WC and et al. (34)	2007	1	No	2
25	Lin CH and et al. (35)	2007	1	Yes	2
26	Saxena AK and et al. (2)	2008	1	No	2
27	Pueyo C and et al. (36)	2009	1	No	3A
28	Sarin YK and et al. (37)	2010	1	No	3A
29	Gudi SN and et al. (38)	2011	1	Yes	3A
30	Deshmukh SD and et al. (7)	2012	1	Yes	2
31	Chouikh t and et al. (10)	2014	1	No	3A

In our experience, we reported a case of newborn with intestinal occlusion where a typical Type 3 atresia with intrauterine intussusception (Figure 1) [10] was found, which may suggest, according to Lmai [18] that the intussusception came after the atresia.

The primary lesion may be the subsequent interference of the intestinal blood supply inducing the intestinal atresia, intussusception of distal segment came after. Histologic study classifies intrauterine intussusception in Types A and B [19].

In Type A the intussuscepted bowel would be located at the distal blind end with good preservation of bowel structure (probably owing to a slight amount of blood supply), as found in the histological analysis of our specimen case.

In Type B, the intussuscepted bowel would be found outside the distal blind end, and it would be necrosed and almost reabsorbed with a typical aspect of Type 2 ileal atresia.

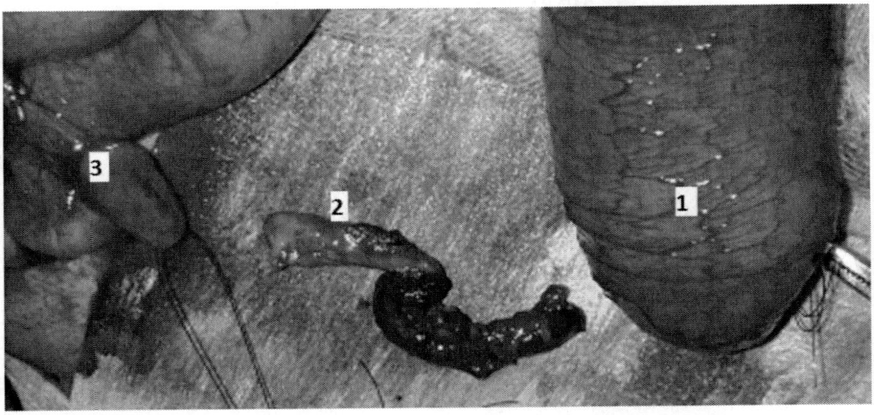

1. Proximal distended ileon
2. Invaginated Segment after reduction of the intussusception
3. Distal ileal Segment that contained the invaginated part

Figure 1. Intra Uterine Intussusception with intestinal atresia.

A definitive preoperative diagnosis may be difficult, if not impossible. Though the usual presentation is that of neonatal intestinal obstruction, and features of peritonitis are usually absent, dilated proximal bowel may perforate and lead to pneumoperitoneum.

The diagnosis is usually made at surgery or more commonly at histopathological examination [3, 20]

References

[1] Price KJ, Roberton NR, Pearse RG. Intussusception in preterm infants. *Arch. Dis. Child.* 1993;68:41-2.

[2] Saxena AK, Van Tuil CV. Intrauterine intussusception in the etiology of jejunal atresia. *Dig. Surg.* 2008; 25:187.

[3] Reed DN Jr, Polley TZ Jr, Rees MA. Jejunal atresia secondary to intrauterine intussusception, presenting as acute perforation. *Can. J. Surg.* 1987;30:203-4.

[4] Millar AJM, Rode HR, Cywes S. Intestinal atresia and stenosis. *In*: Ashcraft KW, Murphy JP, Sharp RJ, Sigalet DL, Snyder CL, editors. Pediatric Surgery. 3rd ed. Philadelphia: WB Saunders; 2000. p. 406-24.

[5] Louw JH, Barnard CN. Congenital intestinal atresia: observation on its origin. *Lancet* 1955;2:1065e7.

[6] Laufman H, Martin WB, Method H. Observations in strangulation obstruction, the fate of sterile devascularized intestine in the peritoneal cavity. *Arch. Surg.* 1949;59:550e64.

[7] De Luca U, Esposito C, Porreca A. Intrauterine intussusception as a cause of ileal atresia occurring late during pregnancy. *Eur. J. Pediatr. Surg.* 1995;5:116e8.

[8] Komuro H, Hori T, Amagai T, Hirai M. The etiologic role of intrauterine volvulus and intussusception in jejunoileal atresia. *J. Pediatr. Surg.* 2004;39: 1812e4.

[9] Todani T, Tabuchi K, Tanaka S. Intestinal atresia due to intrauterine intussusception: analysis of 24 cases in Japan. *J. Pediatr. Surg.* 1975;10:445e51.

[10] Taieb Chouikh, Awatef Charieg, Chaima Mrad ,Sofiene Ghorbel and al: Intestinal atresia caused by intrauterine intussusception: A case report and literature review: *J. Ped. Surg. Case Reports* 2 (2014) 203e205

[11] Gündo_gdu HZ, Senocak ME. Intrauterine intussusception due to Meckel's diverticulum as a cause of ileal atresia: analysis of 2 cases. *Eur. J. Pediatr. Surg.* 1996;6:52e4.

[12] Réguerre Y, de Dreuzy O, Boithias C, Lacaze-Masmonteil T. An unknown etiology of fetal ascites: acute intestinal intussusception. *Arch. Pediatr.* 1997;4: 1197e9.

[13] Kilic N, Kiristioglu I, Kirkpinar A, Dogruyol H. A very rare cause of intestinal atresia intrauterine intussusception due to Meckel's diverticulum. *Acta Paediatr.* 2003;92:756e7.

[14] Shimotake T, Go S, Tsuda T, Iwai N. Ultrasonographic detection of intrauterine intussusception resulting in ileal atresia complicated by meconium peritonitis. *Pediatr. Surg. Int.* 2000;16:43e4.

[15] Shyu MK, Shih J-C, Lee H-N, et al. Correlation of prenatal ultrasound and postnatal outcome in meconium peritonitis. *Fetal. Diagn. Ther.* 2003;18: 255e61.

[16] Wang NL, Yeh ML, Chang PY, Sheu JC, Chen CC, Lee HC, et al. Prenatal and neonatal intussusception. *Pediatr. Surg. Int.* 1998;13:232-6.

[17] Grosfeld JL, Ballantine TV, Shoemaker R Operative management of intestinal atresia and stenosis based on pathologic findings. *J. Pediatr. Surg.* (1979) 14(3): 368-375.

[18] Imai Y, Nishijima E, Muraji T, Hashimoto K, Hayashi Y, Itoh H. Fusion of intussusceptum and intussuscipiens in intrauterine intussusception a rare

[19] Hayashida Y, Ikeda K, Hashimoto N. Histological study of intestinal atresia due to intrauterine intussusception. Z Kinderchir 1984;39:106e9

[20] Rattan KN, Singh Y, Sharma A, Pandit SK, Malik V. Intrauterine intussusception--a cause for ileal atresia. *Indian J. Pediatr.* 2000;67:851-2.

[21] Aubert D, Jung JL, Pageaut G, Gille P. Intestinal atresia after intrauterine intussusception. *Ann. Pediatr.* (Paris) 1982;29:140e1.

[22] Pavri DR, Marshall DG, Armstrong RF, Gorodzinsky FP. Intrauterine intussusception: case report and literature review. *Can. J. Surg.* 1983;26:376e8.

[23] Woodall DL, Birken GA, Williamson K, Lobe TE. Isolated fetal-neonatal abdominal ascites: a sign of intrauterine intussusception. *J. Pediatr. Surg.* 1987; 22:506e7.

[24] Brinson RA, Goldsmith JP. Nonimmune hydrops fetalis associated with intrauterine intussusception. *J. Perinatol.* 1988 Summer;8: 225e7.

[25] Adejuyigbe O, Odesanmi WO. Intrauterine intussusception causing intestinal atresia. *J. Pediatr. Surg.* 1990;25:562e3.

[26] Akgür F, Tanyel FC, Uner H, Büyükpamukçu N, Hiçsönmez A. Intrauterine intussusception: a rare cause of ileal atresia which can lead to confusion in diagnosis. *Turk. J. Pediatr.* 1991;33:55e8.

[27] Kelly SB, Singh MP. Intrauterine intussusception and ileal atresia presenting as acute perforation. *Acta. Paediatr. Scand.* 1991;80:1233e4.

[28] Das PC, Radhakrishna K, Rao PL. Intrauterine intussusception as a cause of intestinal atresia. *Indian Pediatr.* 1992;29:1639e41.

[29] Zijlmans CW, Nabben FA. [Intrauterine invagination in a newborn infant]. *Tijdschr Kindergeneeskd* 1993;61:191e4.

[30] Gündogdu HZ, Senocak ME. Intrauterine intussusception due to Meckel's diverticulum as a cause of ileal atresia: analysis of 2 cases. *Eur. J. Pediatr. Surg.* 1996;6:52e4.
[31] Machmouchi M, Hatoum CA. [Prenatal intestinal invagination. Presentation of a case and review of the literature]. *J. Med. Liban* 2000;48:42e4.
[32] Mcheik JN, Levard G. [Intrauterine intussusception causing intestinal atresia during pregnancy]. *Arch. Pediatr.* 2003;10:230e1.
[33] Yang JI, Kim HS, Chang KH, Hong J. Intrauterine intussusception presenting as fetal ascites at prenatal ultrasonography. *Am. J. Perinatol.* 2004;21:241e6.
[34] Huang WC, Wang CH, Yuh YS, Chen YH. A rare type of ileal atresia due to intrauterine intussusception. *Eur. J. Pediatr.* 2007;166:1177e8.
[35] Lin CH, Wu SF, Lin WC, Chen AC. Meckel's diverticulum induced intrauterine intussusception associated with ileal atresia complicated by meconium peritonitis. *J. Formos. Med. Assoc.* 2007;106:495e8.
[36] Pueyo C, Maldonado J, Royo Y, Skrabski RA. Intrauterine intussusception: a rare cause of intestinal atresia. *J. Pediatr. Surg.* 2009;44:2028e30.
[37] Sarin YK. Intrauterine intussusception causing ileal atresia. *APSP J. Case Rep.* 2010;1:18.
[38] Gudi SN, Bhanuprakash MR, Suneetha V, Prasanna N. Meconium pseudocyst and ileal atresia secondary to intrauterine intussusception. *J. Obstet. Gynaecol. India* 2011;61:562e4.

In: Intussusception and Bowel Obstruction
Editor: Rosie Miller
ISBN: 978-1-63482-703-4

Chapter 5

Laparoscopic Treatment of Intussusception

Philip E. George[1,*], MD, and Edward Chin[2,†], MD, FACS
[1]PGY1 Surgical Resident, Icahn School of Medicine at Mount Sinai, NY, US
[2]Associate Professor of Surgery
Surgical Director, Gastrointestinal Motility Center
Surgical Director, Living Kidney Donor Program
Icahn School of Medicine at Mount Sinai, NY, US

Abstract

Small bowel obstructions are one of the most common indications for surgical intervention for patients presenting to the Emergency Room in the United States. Causes for small bowel obstruction can be divided into several categories: Extraluminal, Intrinsic, and intraluminal causes. The most common cause for the occurrence of an obstruction is adhesions secondary to prior surgeries. Delayed treatment or non-response of an obstruction to medical therapy could potentially lead to perforation, sepsis and ultimately death. Intussusception, or telescoping of the intestine, is a more rare diagnosis, but the natural history is very similar to small bowel obstruction. Prompt diagnosis and initial empiric therapy

* Philip.george@mountsinai.org.
† Edward.Chin@mountsinai.org.

are critical in the management of both conditions. Treatment for both of these processes is at first non-surgical, however worsening of the patients clinic horizon will ultimately necessitate surgical intervention. Historically, general surgeons would perform a laparotomy in order to access the bowel for adhesiolysis. In the last several decades with the advent and improvement of laparoscopic methods, there has been a paradigm shift to diagnostic and therapeutic laparoscopy which is now currently preferred by most academic surgeons. Recent literature shows that minimally invasive techniques are becoming the gold standard for most gastrointestinal surgical procedures, citing reduced length of stay and improved pain control with similar rates of success. In this book chapter, we examine the diagnosis, etiology, pathophysiology and treatment modalities for both small bowel obstruction and intussusception of the small bowel, focusing on minimally invasive surgical options. This is a compilation of the most up to date information on diagnosis and management as well as a review of the current literature regarding safety and efficacy of the least invasive surgical techniques.

Introduction

Intussusception is still a major cause of morbidity and mortality in patients with small bowel obstruction. This presents most frequently in the pediatric population such as after a viral gastroenteritis, but could present in adults in relation to a possible underlying malignancy. Intussusception is defined as a telescoping of one segment of small bowel through another segment. By classical nomenclature the intussusceptum is the prolapsing bowel, and the intussuscipiens is the small bowel encircling the prolapsed bowel.

Between the 1300s-1700s, the only described cases of intussusception were in autopsies [1]. In early medical literature non-operative treatment was the only method of reduction in most patient models. In 1864, Dr. David Grieg, a surgeon from Edinburgh used a bellows as a method of reduction, and in the years following had been a proponent of non-invasive pneumatic flow devices for treatment. Other non-surgical methods have involved air or liquid enemas, oral or topical medications, manual reduction, and even non-contemporary methods such as electricity or ingestion of heavy metals. The role of laparoscopy in the adult population might be straightforward considering the need for possible resection, but in the pediatric population the utility has been questioned [2].

The natural history of intussusception follows a linear path. During normal peristalsis there is rhythmically moving adjacent segments of small or large bowel. If a mass exists along the wall or lumen of the bowel, then that proximal segment presses against it and with enough time and constant pressure (the same mechanism by which it can be reduced) that section of the bowel develops into an intussusceptum. The outward pressure exerted by the mass or lesion on its outer carrier bowel allows the inner bowel to maintain its position. The intussusceptum carries its mesentery along with it and itself becomes entrapped between layers of bowel. The venous network becomes congested and causes an increased level of pressure on the surrounding arterial network. Eventually vascular compromise can cause wall necrosis, perforation, leading to chemical and bacterial peritonitis and even death. This is similar to most other causes of bowel obstruction in that the urgent evaluation and treatment can prevent bowel resection.

Intussusception in the pediatric population has been defined in the literature for decades, but both the treatment and diagnostic algorithms have changed over the same time period. At first, diagnosis was made using injected barium enema, which then migrated to a safer water-based contrast medium. Along with the clinical exam and classic story of "currant-jelly stool," diagnosis can be performed in a quick and consistent manner. The use of ultrasound for diagnosis is also becoming commonplace as well as with the assistance of non-surgical reduction [2]. Where surgery used to be the mainstay for management, most centers have defined intussusception as a non-surgically managed issue [3, 4].

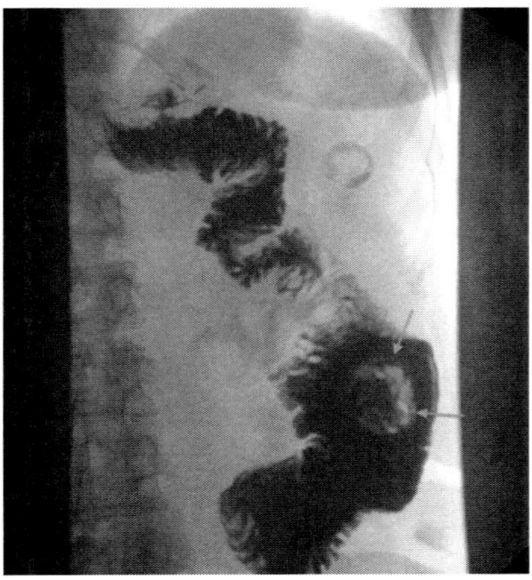

Figure 1. Contrast enema showing a filling defect at the arrows.

Diagnosis of the intussusception can be done with barium enema, GI series follow through, ultrasonography, computed tomography, or clinical exam. Studies showing any filling defect through a portion of bowel with portions of the bowel coming in and out of place could be associated with intussusception (Figure 1).

The advancement of Computed Tomography, reduction in its radiation dose as well as its use to evaluate non-specific abdominal has led to increased diagnosis of intussusception using this technique. Visualization of the anatomy of the abdomen grants CT scanning a distinct advantage in a patient with an uncertain diagnosis. A very specific pathognomonic would be the *target sign*, which showcases the two distinct and separate layers of bowel wall inside of one another (Figure 2-3).

After intussusception is diagnosed an attempt is first made to use an air-pressure enema for reduction [5]. After an attempt and failure, a laparoscopic approach is attempted. Failure of enema reduction has been implicated in roughly 10-20% of all cases and at that time mandates surgical intervention [6, 7]. Intussusceptions involving ileo-ileal segments are most often amenable to laparoscopic reduction, but any segment involving more distal parts of the colon might more likely be able to be reduced using an open approach [8].

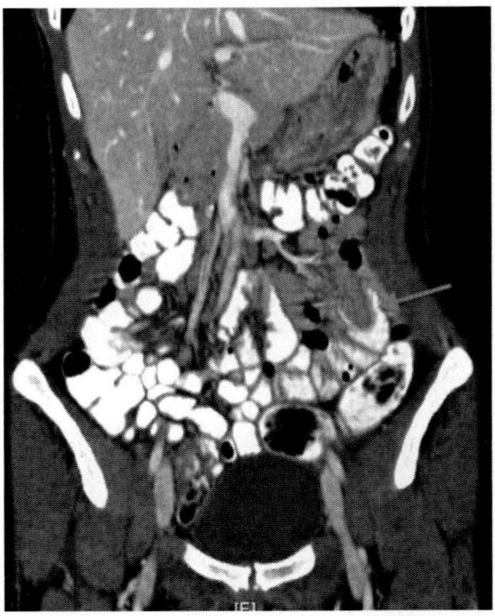

Figure 2. Jejuno-jejunal intussusception shown in coronal view (Arrow denoting tip of invagination of bowel).

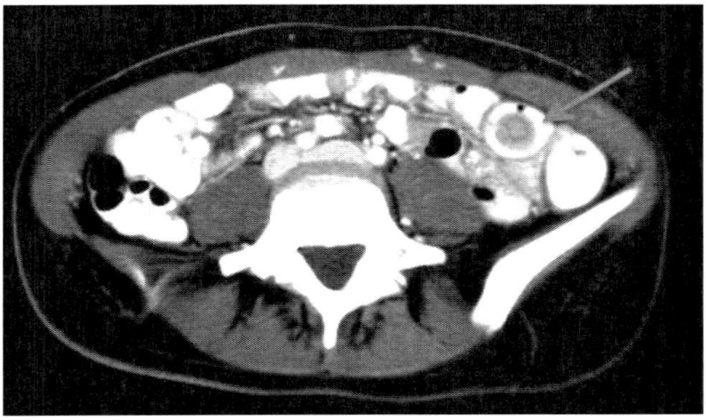

Figure 3. Target sign of Jejuno-jejunal intussusception shown in axial view. (Arrow denoting separated layers of bowel, causing target formation).

Pre-Procedure

For most cases, a preoperative bowel regimen is unnecessary, especially in patients who are experiencing sepsis secondary to peritonitis, and pre-operative antibiotics are unnecessary for cases without perforation. Routine use of nasogastric tube is indicated for gastric and upper GI decompression to reduce the incidence of vomiting and aspiration during intubation.

Positioning and Trocar Placement

Positioning of the patient involves the supine position with the surgeon positioned at the patients left with the assistant surgeon either opposite of the primary surgeon or off to the primary surgeons side holding camera. One 5mm port is inserted into the umbilicus using a Veress needle under direct visualization. Pneumoperitoneum is then induced with carbon dioxide at a flow rate to the surgeon's discretion. Then a 4mm 30 degree scope is inserted and used for visualization of the bowel.

Depending on the location of the pathology, a 2mm trocar is inserted into the left lower quadrant or right lower quadrant using laparoscopic visualization. Instrumentation can be done with either 2mm or 5mm instruments. Instruments that are 2mm are more susceptible to serosal tears since they are unable to provide sufficient force of retraction. The surgeon must keep in mind spontaneous reduction of the intussusception might have already occurred at the point of visualization whether due to continued peristalsis or by pneumoperitoneum.

For ileo-cecal intussusceptions, a 2mm or 5mm grasper is used with the surgeon's left hand to grab firm hold of the cecum. Preferences could be either to use a Babcock or a bowel grasper. The grasper is clamped onto the entirety of the small bowel wall and extended onto the small bowel mesentery and firm pressure is applied. The bowel should be distracted slowly in opposite directions in order to give time for areas of edema to shift. After constant force is applied for a long enough period of time the bowel should give way. This technique can be applied to ileo-ileal or jejuno-ileal intussusceptions as well, being sure to keep in mind the size of the grasper and that you must distribute the pressure evenly along the entirety of the grasped bowel wall.

In some institutions, a rectal Foley catheter can be placed cautiously, attached to saline at high flow, and manipulated by a non-sterile surgical team member or staff member in order to offer counter-pressure and assistance in reduction [9].

If the surgeon is unable to reduce with 2mm instruments, the 2mm trocar sites can be exchanged for 5mm sites and 5mm instruments can be used.

The algorithm then extends to pursuit of treatment after laparoscopic treatment has failed or if decompensation is noted. One method many surgeons use intraoperative before the decision is made to convert to open is to use an intraoperative enema that is then placed under laparoscopic control. However if during the procedure, any signs of bowel necrosis or mass is seen forming a lead point, the decision is universally to convert to open to complete the remainder of the procedure which involves resection of the affected segments.

Post-Procedure Care

After completion of the procedure, lidocaine should be infiltrated into the trocar sites. Post-operative pain control can be managed with Tylenol. Most surgeons feel comfortable discharging on post-operative day number 3 if the diagnosis was idiopathic in nature.

In patients who solely went reduction of the idiopathic intussusception, resumption of diet can occur on post-operative day #1, but for patients undergoing resection it is felt as though a slower return to diet is more appropriate. This can occur when patient is passing flatus or on post-operative day #3, whichever the surgeon feels more comfortable with.

Intussusception in the Adult Patient

Intussusception in the adult population is a rare event that has been described in the literature since 1674. It can be caused from a mass effect in the bowel wall, increase in peristalsis, or any irritation of the bowel lumen. While only 1-2 percent of small bowel obstruction in adults are due to intussusception, roughly 50 percent of intussusception is due to malignancy [10, 11]. In one medical center over a span of 16 years, out of a total of 17,000 patients treated with surgery for small bowel obstruction, only 44 were attributed to intussusception [12].

The optimal treatment for intussusception in adults is based off of several factors which include prior surgeries, clinical status, and also ability to undergo invasive surgery [13]. At most medical institutions it is always believed to try and undergo resection without reduction since up to 24 percent of enteric intussusception are due to malignancy and about 50 percent of colonic cases are due to malignancy. This methodology of treating with resection prior to reduction is especially important since most cases are discovered upon exploratory surgery [14, 15]. It is advised by many groups that operative reduction in the adult should not even be attempted as tumor seeding the peritoneum or disseminating is possible [16]. When the definitive cause of the intussusception can be traced back to trauma or it is caused intra-operatively, the consensus is that reduction can be performed safely.

Discussion

Laparoscopy is an effective tool the general or pediatric surgeon can use for idiopathic or pathologic intussusception that has a solid role as both a diagnostic and therapeutic tool. While not replacing the initial non-operatively enema reduction in the pediatric population, it has actually been the first line diagnostic and treatment tool for adult patients, given that a lead point is the most common underlying cause.

A number of techniques are being described at several medical centers using laparoscopy for the reduction of intussusception that avoid the use of a laparotomy. One of these techniques is the Chinese Fan Spread technique pioneered by Chui et al. [17] The technique involves standard laparoscopy using 5mm instruments to walk the bowel towards the point of intussusception. The actual technique comes from using crossed 5mm bowel graspers and slowly opening the angle between them to distract the adjacent segments of bowel away from each other. A fenestrated grasper was used in this study for its ability to apply strong traction during the reduction technique as well as distribute force to reduce incidences of bowel perforation. After reduction, as is standard practice, bowel is still examined for presence of a lead point or other pathology. The theory of using a fulcrum as a method of establishing reduction seems to have worked in this surgeon group. Twelve patients of fourteen were able to be reduced with the Chinese Fan Spread technique, while the other 2 had to undergo laparotomy. The patients who had to undergo laparotomy underwent resection since the bowel could not be manually reduced. This technique shows an effectiveness of 86% for reduction of intussusception after failed air enema. No complications were noted in this small patient population, so the technique must be applied broadly in order to interpret possible complications.

Laparotomy has for the most part been replaced by laparoscopy in the developed world for the first surgical step in a patient presumed to have intussusception that failed non-surgical therapy. In a single study comparison of primary laparotomy vs laparoscopy for intussusception in pediatric patients, length of stay was significantly reduced for the laparoscopic group (3.00 +/- 1.31 days) compared to the open group (4.52 +/- 1.98) [9]. However complications and operating time were not significantly different. Cost however was reduced in the laparoscopic group. These results have been reflected in multiple other studies. As well as incorporating the aesthetic scar, the length of hospital stay and cost should be enough incentive for most hospital centers to adopt a solely primary laparoscopic approach to this issue.

In a study performed in Egypt on a group of pediatric patients with intussusception, a total of 20 patients were evaluated and treated after continued symptoms from failed hydrostatic reduction [18]. At laparoscopy a total of 8 patients had the intussusception reduced at laparoscopy and 6 other patients had successful reduction using intra-operative enema reduction. The other 6 patients had to undergo laparotomy for reduction. A total of 70% of patients with failed enema reduction were able to be reduced with laparoscopy.

In conclusion, laparoscopy is becoming a very effective method at reducing intussusception in the pediatric population and thereby avoiding the need for laparotomy. In the adult population it is a useful diagnostic and therapeutic tool to evaluate for lead points as well as aiding in resection. New laparoscopic techniques are being developed and might be more effective than conventional technique, but even conventional laparoscopy is a safe and effective technique for reduction or resection of adult or pediatric intussusceptions.

References

[1] Frush DP, Zheng, J, McDermott, VG, Bisset III, GS. Nonoperative treatment of intussusception: historical perspective. *AJR* 1995;165:1066-1070.

[2] van der Laan M, Bax NMA, van der Zee DC. The role of laparoscopy in the management of childhood intussusception. *Surgical Endoscopy* 2001;15(4):373-376.

[3] Lain AH, Firman K. Ultrasound of intussusception with lead points. *Australas Radiol* 1991;35:343-345.

[4] Pierro A, Donnell SC, Paraskevopoulou C, Carty H, Lloyd DA. Indications for laparotomy after hydrostatic reduction for intussusception. *J Pediatr Surg* 1993;28:1154-1157.

[5] Guo JZ, Ma XY, Zhou QH. Results of air pressure enema reduction of intussusception: 6,396 cases in 13 years. *J Pediatr Surg* 1986;21:1201–1203.

[6] G.S. Bisset, D.R. Kirks. Intussusception in infants and children: diagnosis and therapy. *Radiology* 1998;168:141–145.

[7] S.O. Choi, W.H. Park, S.K. Woo. Ultrasound-guided water enema: an alternative method to nonoperative treatment for childhood intussusception. *J. Pediatr. Surg.* 1994;29:498–500.

[8] Hay SA, Kabesh AA, Soliman HA et al. Idiopathic intussusception: the role of laparoscopy. *J Pediatr Surg* 1999;34:577–578.

[9] Kia KF, Mony VK, Drongowski RA, Golladay ES, Gieger JD, Hirschl RB, Coran AG, Teitelbaum DH. Laparoscopic vs open surgical approach for intussusception requiring operative intervention. *J Pediatr Surg* 2005;40(1):281-284.

[10] Solazzo M, Chiodini S, Puccio F. Laparoscopic Surgery For Adult Bowel Intussusception: Report Of A Case. *The Internet Journal of Surgery* 2004;6(2).

[11] Honjo H, Mike M, Kusanagi H, Kano N. Adult Intussusception: A Retrospective Review. *World J Surgery.* 2015;39(1):134-138.

[12] Weilbaecher D, Bolin JA, Hearn D. Intussusception in adults: review of 160 patients. *Am J Surg* 1971;121:531–535.

[13] Felix EL, Cohen MH, Bernstein AD. Adult intussusception: patient report of recurrent intussusception and review of the literature. *Am J Surg* 1976;131:758–761.

[14] Azar T, Berger DL. Adult intussusception. *Ann Surg* 1997;226:134–138.

[15] Agha FP. Intussusception in adults. *AJR Am J Roentgenol* 1986;146:527–531.

[16] Begos DG, Sandor A, Modlin IM. The diagnosis and management of adult intussusception. *The American Journal of Surgery* 1997;173(2):88-94.

[17] Chui CH, Ong LY, Chua JH, Yap TL. "Chinese Fan Spread" Distraction Technique of Laparoscopic Reduction of Intussusception. *JSLS* 2007;11(2):238-241.

[18] Elkader AH , Elshafei E, Safaan H. Laparoscopic Assisted Pneumatic Reduction of Intussusception in Infants and Children. Annals of Pediatric Surgery 2009;5(2):98-100.

In: Intussusception and Bowel Obstruction
Editor: Rosie Miller
ISBN: 978-1-63482-703-4

Chapter 6

Afferent Loop Obstruction

***K. Blouhos*[1,*], *K. A. Boulas*[1,†], *K. Tsalis*[2,‡] *and A. Hatzigeorgiadis*[1,§]**
[1]Department of General Surgery, General Hospital of Drama, Drama, Greece
[2]D' Surgical Department, "G. Papanikolaou" Hospital, Medical School, Aristotle University of Thessaloniki, Thessaloniki, Greece

Abstract

Afferent loop obstruction is a purely mechanical complication that infrequently occurs following construction of a gastrojejunostomy. The operations most commonly associated with this complication are gastrectomy with Billroth II or Roux-en-Y reconstruction, and pancreaticoduodenectomy with conventional loop or Roux-en-Y reconstruction. Etiology of afferent loop obstruction includes: (a)

* Konstantinos Blouhos MD, MSc, PhD - HPB-GI Surgeon - Staff Surgeon - Department of General Surgery, General Hospital of Drama, Drama, Greece: kostasblu@hotmail.com.
† Corresponding author: Konstantinos A. Boulas, MD, MSc, Department of General Surgery, General Hospital of Drama, End of Hippokratous Street, 66100 Drama, Greece. Tel: +306937265675; Fax: +302513501559; E-mail: katerinantwna@hotmail.com.
‡ Konstantinos Tsalis MD, PhD - HPB Surgeon - Professor of Surgery and Chairman - D' Surgical Department, "G. Papanikolaou" Hospital, Medical School, Aristotle University of Thessaloniki, Thessaloniki, Greece: ctsalis@yahoo.gr.
§ Anestis Hatzigeorgiadis MD, MSc, PhD - Chairman - Department of General Surgery, General Hospital of Drama, Drama, Greece: ahatz@otenet.gr.

entrapment, compression and kinking by postoperative adhesions; (b) internal herniation, volvulus and intussusception; (c) scarring and stenosis due to ulceration at the gastrojejunostomy site and radiation enteritis; (d) cancer recurrence; (e) enteroliths, bezoars and foreign bodies. Acute afferent loop obstruction is associated with complete obstruction of the afferent loop and represents a surgical emergency, whereas chronic afferent loop obstruction is associated with partial obstruction. Abdominal MDCT is the diagnostic study of choice. CT appearance of the obstructed afferent loop is a C-shaped, fluid-filled tubular mass located in the midline between the abdominal aorta and the superior mesenteric artery with valvulae conniventes projecting into the lumen. The cornerstone of treatment is surgery. Surgery includes: (a) adhesiolysis and reconstruction for benign causes; (b) by-pass or excision and reconstruction for malignant causes. However, endoscopic and transhepatic or direct percutaneous interventions for enteral stent insertion have the principal role in the in the management of malignant and radiation-induced obstruction. Nevertheless, considerable limitations exist as a former Roux-en-Y reconstruction limits endoscopic access to the afferent loop and percutaneous approaches for enteric stenting and tube enterostomy have only been reported in the literature as isolated cases.

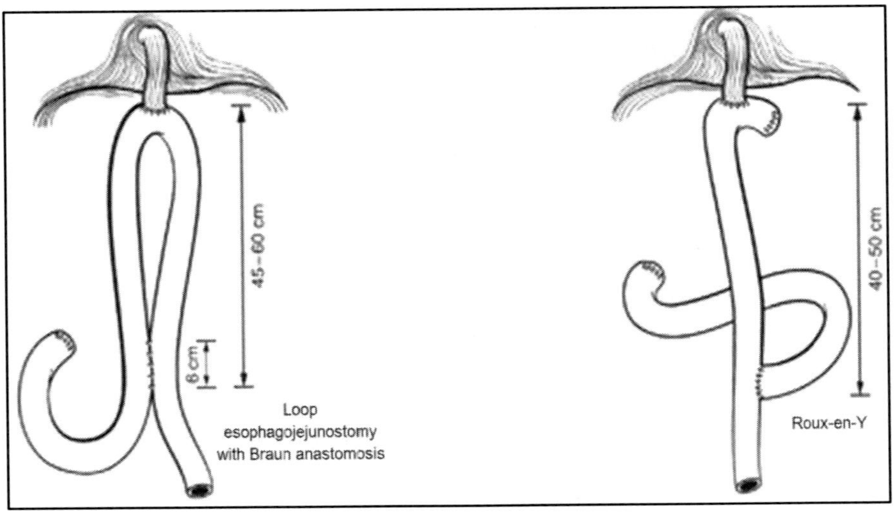

(a)

Figure 1. (Continued).

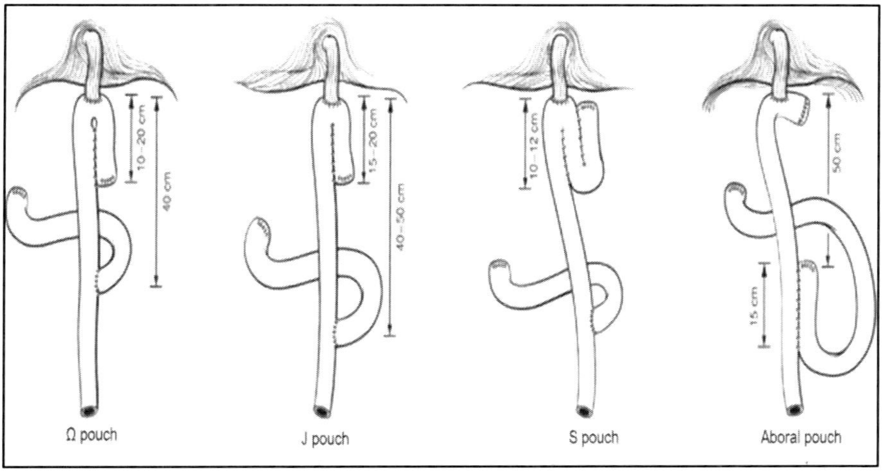

(b)

Figure 1. Schematic presentantion of total gastrectomy with (a) loop esophagojejunostomy and simple Roux-en-Y reconstruction, and (b) pouch Roux-en-Y reconstruction.

Definitions

Creation of a gastrojejunostomy leaves a segment of proximal small bowel, most commonly consisting of duodenum and proximal jejunum, lying upstream from the gastrojejunostomy. This limb of intestine conducts bile, pancreatic juices, and other proximal intestinal secretions toward the gastrojejunostomy and is termed the afferent loop [1]. Afferent loop obstruction (ALO) is a purely mechanical complication that infrequently occurs following construction of a gastrojejunostomy. The operations most commonly associated with this complication include total gastrectomy with loop esophagojejunostomy and simple or pouch Roux-en-Y reconstruction (Figure 1), partial gastrectomy with Billroth II and Roux-en-Y reconstruction (Figure 2), and pancreaticoduodenectomy with conventional loop and Roux-en-Y reconstruction (Figure 3) performed for treatment of benign and malignant causes [2].

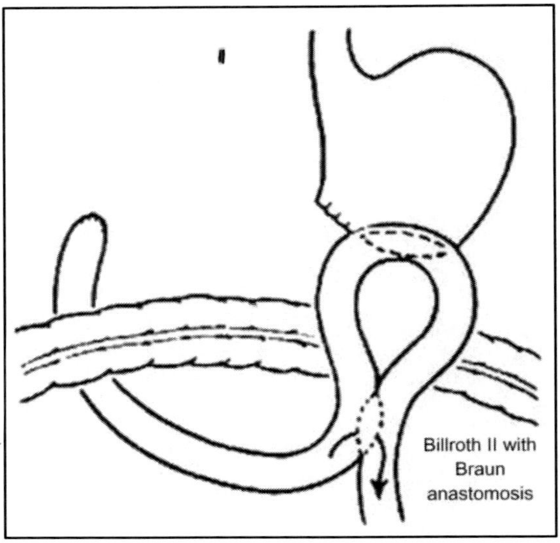

(a)

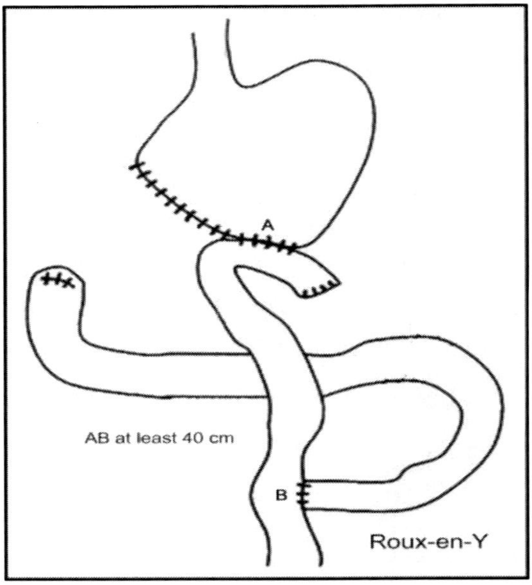

(b)

Figure 2. Schematic presentantion of partial gastrectomy with (a) Billroth II and (b) Roux-en-Y reconstruction.

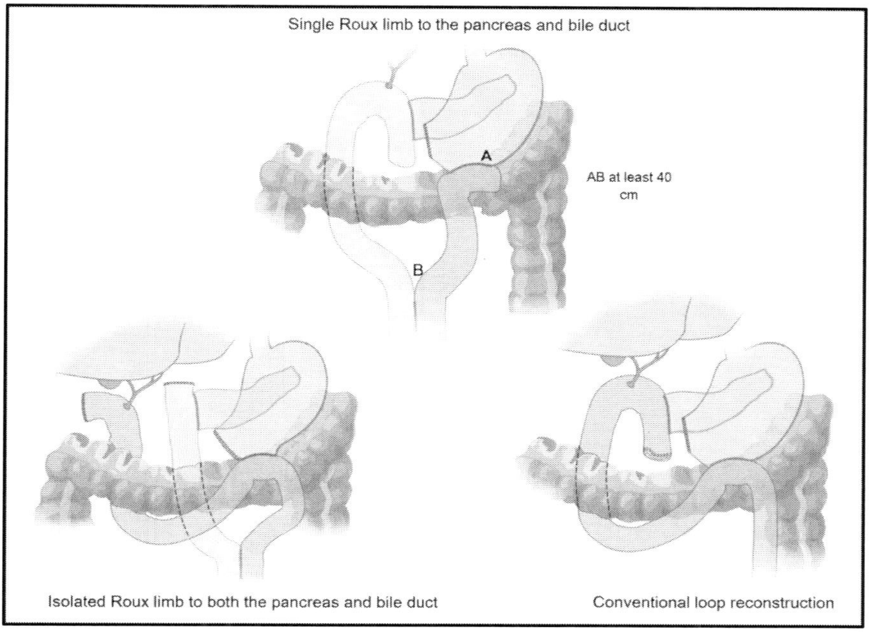

Figure 3. Schematic presentantion of pancreaticoduodenectomy with conventional loop and Roux-en-Y reconstruction.

Etiology

Causes of ALO include: (1) Entrapment, compression and kinking of the afferent loop by postoperative adhesions [3]; (2) Internal herniation, volvulus and intussusception of the afferent loop [4]; (3) Scarring due to marginal ulceration of the gastrojejunostomy [5]; (4) Locoregional recurrence (lymph nodes, peritoneum, gastric remnant, anastomotic sites) [6]; (5) Radiation enteritis [7]; and (6) Enteroliths, bezoars and foreign bodies impacted in the afferent loop [8]. However, it is useful to classify obstruction according to the benign or malignant nature of the obstructing lesion in order to highlight the presentantion, natural history and management strategy of ALO (Table 1). Risk factors for ALO include: (a) Redundant (longer than 30-40 cm) and antecolic afferent loop which are more prone to kinking, volvulus, and entrapment by adhesions; and (b) Improperly closed mesocolic defects which predispose to internal herniation of the retrocolic afferent loop [9].

Table 1. Classification of afferent loop obstructions and management strategy

Causes			Management
Benign	Intraluminal	Foreign bodies Bezoar Enteroliths Intussusception	Surgery
	Intramural	Gastrojejunostomy ulceration	
	Extrinsic	Adhesions Volvulus Internal hernia	
Malignant Radiation enteritis	Recurrence	Gastric remnant Anastomotic sites Lymph nodes Peritoneum Carcinomatosis	Endoscopy for enteral stenting Transhepatic or direct percutaneous interventions for enteral stenting By-pass surgery Excision of the former afferent loop and reconstruction

Incidence

The incidence of ALO after distal gastrectomy with Billroth II or Roux-en-Y reconstruction has been reported to be 0.3–1.0% [10]. The incidence of ALO is similar in open and laparoscopic surgery although there are several specific predisposing factors for ALO following laparoscopic gastrectomy such as partial omentectomy and antecolic anastomosis. Kim et al. in their retrospective cohort study, reported 4 (1.01%) patients who developed ALO among 386 gastric cancer patients submitted to laparoscopic distal gastrectomy with Billroth II reconstruction. The interval between the initial gastrectomy and the operation for ALO ranged from 4 to 540 days (median 33 days). The causes of ALO included adhesions in 2 patients and internal herniation in 2 patients. All patients recovered following the emergency operations [11]. Aoki et al. in their retrospective cohort study, reported 4

(0.2%) patients who developed ALO among 1908 gastric cancer patients submitted to distal gastrectomy with Roux-en-Y reconstruction. The causes of the ALO included internal herniation in two patients, adhesions in one patient, and peritoneal recurrence in one patient. The interval between the initial gastrectomy and emergency operation for ALO ranged from 3 weeks to 2 years (median 5 months). All patients recovered following emergency operations, and none died of this complication [12].

There are limited data on the incidence of ALO after pancreaticoduodenectomy, especially among long-term pancreatic cancer survivors (> 2 years). In one of the few studies in the literature, Pannala et al. evaluated the incidence of ALO in pancreatic cancer patients submitted to pancreaticoduodenectomy. Pannala et al. in their retrospective cohort study, reported 24 (13%) patients who developed ALO among 186 pancreatic cancer patients treated with PD. Median time to diagnosis was 1.2 years (range 0.03-12.3 years). Obstruction was primarily caused by recurrent pancreatic cancer in 8 patients (33%) and radiation enteritis of the afferent loop in 9 patients (38%) [13].

Pathophysiology

Symptoms associated with ALO are caused by increased intraluminal pressure and distention due to accumulation of enteric, biliary and pancreatic secretions in the partially or completely obstructed afferent loop. The severity at presentation mainly depends on the degree and duration of obstruction [14]. Acute ALO, which represents a complete obstruction of the afferent loop, can lead to: (a) Closed-loop obstruction. Ischemia and gangrene of the completely obstructed afferent loop with subsequent perforation and peritonitis evolve rapidly; (b) Ascending cholangitis and pancreatitis. Chronic ALO, which represents a partial obstruction of the afferent loop, can lead to: (a) Open-loop obstruction. Although the partially obstructed afferent loop can be decompressed, open-loop obstruction is often complicated by events similar to those seen in closed-loop obstruction; (b) Ascending cholangitis and pancreatitis; and (c) Bacterial overgrowth in the afferent loop. Bacteria deconjugate bile acids, which can lead to steatorrhea, malnutrition, and vitamin B-12 deficiency. Megaloblastic anemia is added to the existing iron deficiency anemia which is a result of bypassing the proximal small bowel and achlorhydria which impairs iron solubility [15].

Presentantion

The primary symptoms of patients with acute ALO are sudden, severe abdominal pain and vomiting. The pain often occurs before associated findings of localized abdominal tenderness and involuntary guarding develop. When physical findings develop, there is a high level of suspicion that the viability of the bowel is compromised. When bowel obstruction (small or large intestine, afferent or efferent loop) is the most likely diagnosis, abdominal pain out of proportion to physical findings represents a surgical emergency. The vomitus is not bilious because the biliary and pancreatic secretions remain trapped in the obstructed afferent loop [16].

Chronic ALO is more difficult to diagnose than acute ALO. Chronic ALO may manifest as periumbilical discomfort, developing 15-30 minutes after eating and often lasting 1 to 4 hours. These patients develop food fear and modify their pattern of eating so that they only consume small quantity of food at any one time. Patients with chronic ALO almost always have a profound weight loss, which raises suspicion of intraabominal malignancy. The progression from open-loop obstruction which is characterized by minor symptoms to closed-loop obstruction which represent a true surgical emergency is unpredictable. Projectile bilious vomiting may occur as the distended afferent loop decompresses forcefully providing rapid relief of symptoms. Chronic ALO with stasis and bacterial overgrowth can be further complicated by steatorrhea, diarrhea, vitamin B-12 and iron deficiency anemia [17].

Physical examination can reveal one or more of the following findings: (1) Upper abdominal distention. An ill-defined mass in the upper abdomen may be palpated which represents the completely obstructed afferent loop; (2) Localized upper abdominal tenderness and involuntary guarding if perforation and peritonitis have occured; (3) Jaundice; and (4) Signs of pancreatitis.

Imaging Studies

Prior to the era of CT, conventional upper gastrointestinal barium studies were used to assess ALO. Two classical findings of ALO were described: (1) Non-filling of the afferent loop; and (2) Retention of barium in the dilated afferent loop for at least 60 minutes. However, several limitations existed as 20% of normal afferent loops were not filled with a barium meal and the underlying cause of obstruction was poorly identified [18]. Currently, CT plays an important role in the diagnosis of ALO. Zissin et al. reported that the characteristic CT appearance of the obstructed afferent loop is a U or C-shaped, fluid-filled, 5.3 cm in average diameter, tubular mass (C-loop sign) located in the midline between the abdominal aorta and the superior mesenteric artery with valvulae conniventes projecting into the lumen (keyboard sign) which can help in the differential diagnosis of pancreatic pseudocysts [19]. Juan et al. reviewed MDCT scans of 22 patients who developed ALO after partial gastrectomy and pancreaticoduodenectomy. The C-loop appearance was present in 22 patients (100%) and the keyboard sign in 21 patients (95%) (Figure 4). There was only 1 patient without the presence of the keyboard sign due to bowel perforation. The maximal diameter of the afferent loop ranged from 3.3 to 5.8 cm [20].

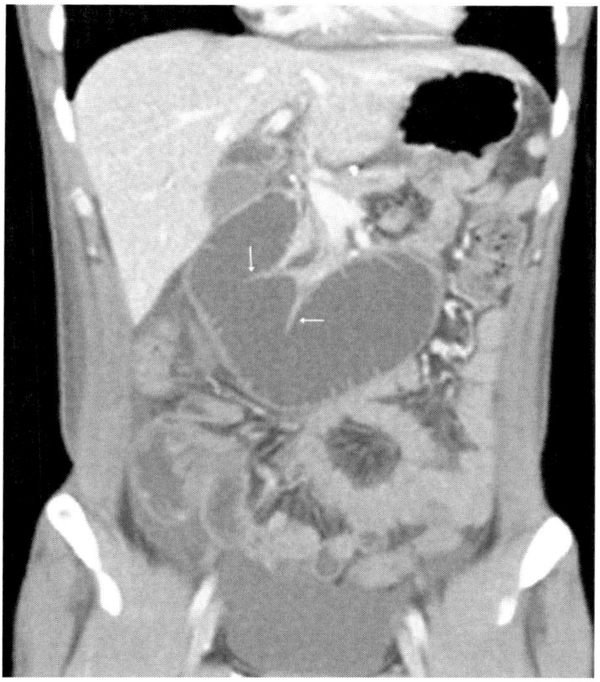

Figure 4. The C-loop and the keyboard sign (arrows).

CT can provide accurate determination of the cause of ALO. CT images should be evaluated for the presence of: (1) the C-loop sign; (2) the keyboard sign; (3) pancreaticobiliary tract dilatation; (4) bowel wall thickening at the anastomotic sites, the afferent and efferent loops; (5) lymphadenopathy, ascites, peritoneal enhancement, and metastatic lesions. Adhesions are suspected when a point of transition from a dilated to a normal-caliber loop is observed without other apparent cause. An internal hernia is suspected when crowding, stretching, and crossover of mesenteric vessels and the whirl sign are observed. Local recurrence and radiation enteritis are suspected when focal and diffuse bowel wall thickening are present, respectively. Carcinomatosis is suspected when ascites and peritoneal enhancement are present and bowel wall thickening around the level of obstruction is absent [21]. Kim et al. reviewed helical CT scans of 18 patients who developed ALO after partial gastrectomy. The presumed cause of obstruction on CT was compared with surgical findings and clinical courses. In all 8 patients who underwent a second operation the cause of afferent loop was correctly suggested on CT. In all 10 patients who were not re-explored, the clinical findings or biopsy indicated recurrent tumor as suggested on CT. The authors concluded that the causes of ALO can be correctly predicted with CT [22].

MRCP or secretin-enhanced MRCP should be added in the diagnostic workup when a pancreaticoduodenectomy is preceded. The incidence of biliary and pancreatic stricture after pancreaticoduodenectomy is 2.6% and 2%, respectively. The patency of the primary hepaticojejunostomy and pancreaticojejunostomy should be thoroughly evaluated because the presence of a stricture can alter management strategy of ALO. Anatomic variants (pancreas divisum, dominant dorsal duct, aberrant ductal communications) and ductal pathology including filling defects, stenosis or obstruction should be recorded [23]. A hepaticojejunostomy stricture is characterized by the presence of a fixed filling defect at the anastomotic site, along with post-obstructive extra- and intra-hepatic ductal dilation. A pancreaticojejunostomy stricture is characterized by the presence of a fixed filling defect at the anastomotic site, along with post-obstructive ductal dilation, side-branch enhancement and/or decreased functional excretion into the jejunal drainage limb [24].

Management

As radiation-induced ALO is an infrequent complication of gastrectomy and pancreaticoduodenectomy, the literature on management of this complication is limited and much of the current knowledge on its management is derived by the accrual of single-institution series. Management strategy

(Table 2) depends on the following three factors: (1) The benign or malignant nature of the obstructing lesion. ALO caused by a benign lesion needs definitive treatment by surgery which includes repair of the primary cause along with a form of afferent loop reconstruction which includes: (a) addition of a Braun anastomosis in a former Billroth II reconstruction; (b) excision of the redundant loop and conversion of Billroth II to Roux-en-Y gastrojejunostomy; (c) excision of the redundant loop and reconstruction of the former Roux-en-Y jejunojejunostomy). ALO caused by a malignant lesion needs either palliative treatment (percutaneous and endoscopic interventions, by-pass surgery) or surgery with curative intent (excision and reconstruction); (2) The site of obstruction. An obstruction at the inframesocolic portion of the afferent loop can be easily reconstructed, whereas an obstruction at the surpramesocolic portion of the afferent loop needs copious mobilization of the supramesocolic segment of the afferent loop through a field of dense adhesions; and (3) The patency of the primary hepaticojejunostomy and pancreaticojejunostomy. ALO in the setting of a preceded pancreatico-duodenectomy may require revision of the hepaticojejunostomy and pancreaticojejunostomy and/or a modified Puestow procedure during reconstruction of the obstructed afferent loop due to an anastomotic stenosis demonstrated in the preoperative secretin-enhanced MRCP [25].

As referred above, surgery has the principal role in the management of benign ALO. On the contrary, more conservative approaches are preferred in the setting of malignant ALO as in the literature there are no data showing differences in survival between patients who submitted to palliative and curative treatment for management of malignant ALO. Endoscopic interventions at the afferent loop for enteral stent insertion (balloon dilation, double-pigtail stents traversing the afferent loop strictured area, balloon dilation and double-pigtail stent placement, afferent loop metal stent placement), the bile duct (biliary balloon dilation and plastic or metal stent placement through ERCP), and the pancreatic duct (pancreatic duct balloon dilation and stent placement through ERCP or EUS-guided rendezvous drainage after unsuccessful ERCP) have a principal role in the management of malignant ALO [26]. In Pannala et al. series, fifteen patients (62%) had an endoscopic intervention for management of malignant ALO after pancreaticoduodenectomy with Billroth II reconstruction for pancreatic cancer. These patients required a median of 2 endoscopic procedures (range 1-17 endoscopic procedures); eleven patients (73%) had clinical and laboratory improvement, two patients (13%) did not improve, and two patients (13%) were lost to follow-up [13]. However, a Roux-en-Y reconstruction limits endoscopic access to the afferent loop [27]. Enteral stenting and ERCP with double-balloon enteroscope in patients with Roux-en-Y anastomosis have only been reported in the literature as small single-institute series [28]. Moreover, transhepatic or direct percutaneous enteral stent insertion for management of ALO have only been reported in the literature as isolated cases [29]. When endoscopic and percutaneous approaches are neither successful nor feasible, redo surgery of becomes inevitable. Re-operative surgery for management of malignant ALO is a difficult undertaking and re-operation itself may be the cause of further morbidity and mortality. Re-operation rates vary from 4% to 11% among small-volume series [30]. When redo surgery is indicated, more conservative surgical approaches in these challenging group of patients, such as by-pass surgery, should be performed. When all the above approaches (percutaneous approach, endoscopic approach, by-pass surgery) fail, excision of the obstructed afferent loop and reconstruction should be considered as a treatment option [31].

Table 2. Management of afferent loop obstructions

Causes		Management	
		Former Billroth II	*Former Roux-en-Y*
Benign	Enteroliths Bezoar Foreign bodies	Adhesiolysis, enterotomy, removal and repair of anastomotic stenosis after preoperative assessment with barium meal in chronic obstruction (Stricturoplasty, addition of Braun anastomosis, conversion to Roux-en-Y)	Adhesiolysis, enterotomy, removal and repair of anastomotic stenosis after preoperative assessment with barium meal in chronic obstruction (Stricturoplasty, revision of the Roux-en-Y reconstruction)
	Intussusce-ption	Manual reduction or enterectomy and conversion to Roux-en-Y	Manual reduction, or enterectomy and revision of the Roux-en-Y reconstruction
	Gastroje-junostomy ulceration	Stricturoplasty or conversion to Roux-en-Y	Stricturoplasty or revision of the Roux-en-Y reconstruction
	Adhesions	Adhesiolysis, Braun anastomosis or excision of redundant loop and conversion to Roux-en-Y	Adhesiolysis, excision of redundant loop and revision of the jejunojejunostomy
	Volvulus	Enterectomy and conversion to Roux-en-Y	Enterectomy and revision of the Roux-en-Y

Causes		Management	
		Former Billroth II	*Former Roux-en-Y* reconstruction
	Internal hernia	Reduction and repair of the defect or reduction, repair of the defect, enterectomy and conversion to Roux-en-Y	Reduction and repair of the defect or reduction, repair of the defect, enterectomy and revision of the Roux-en-Y reconstruction
Malignant Radiation enteritis		Endoscopy (balloon dilation and double-pigtail stents traversing the afferent limb strictured area, afferent limb metal stent placement) By-pass surgery when endoscopy fails Adhesiolysis, mobilization and excision of the former afferent loop, Roux-en-Y reconstruction including construction or revision (in preceded pancreaticoduodenectomy) of HJ and PJ (pancreaticojejuno-jejunostomy if primary PJ has normal patency in preoperative MRCP [31] or revision of the PJ and/or modified Puestow if primary PJ is strictured [32])	Enteral stenting with double-balloon enteroscope Percutaneous approaches for endoluminal stenting By-pass surgery when endoscopy fails Adhesiolysis, mobilization and excision of the former afferent loop, revision of the Roux-en-Y reconstruction including construction or revision (in preceded pancreaticoduodenectomy) of HJ and PJ (pancreaticojejuno-jejunostomy if primary PJ has normal patency in preoperative MRCP [31] or revision of the PJ and/or modified Puestow if primary PJ is strictured [32])

HJ: hepaticojejunostomy, PJ: pancreaticojejunostomy.

References

[1] Woodfield CA, Levine MS (2005) The postoperative stomach. *Eur J Radiol* 53:341-352.

[2] Bolton JS, Conway WC (2011) Postgastrectomy syndromes. *Surg Clin North* 91:1105-1122.

[3] Uchida H, Sakamoto S, Hamano I, Kobayashi M, Kitajima T, Shigeta T, Kanazawa H, Fukuda A, Kasahara M (2014) Urgent living donor liver transplantation for biliary atresia complicated by a strangulated internal hernia at Roux-en Y limb: a case report. *Ann Transplant* 19:149-152.

[4] Lee SY, Lee JC, Yang DH (2013) Early Postoperative Retrograde Jejunojejunal Intussusception after Total Gastrectomy with Roux-en-Y Esophagojejunostomy: A Case Report. *J Gastric Cancer* 13:263-265.

[5] Ballas KD, Rafailidis SE, Konstantinidis HD, Pavlidis TE, Marakis GN, Anagnostara E, Sakadamis AK (2009) Acute afferent loop syndrome: a true emergency. A case report. *Acta Chir Belg* 109:101-103.

[6] Yoshida H, Mamada Y, Taniai N, Mizuguchi Y, Kakinuma D, Ishikawa Y, Nakamura Y, Okuda T, Kiyama T, Tajiri T (2008) Afferent loop obstruction treated by percutaneous transhepatic insertion of an expandable metallic stent. *Hepatogastroenterology* 55:1767-1769..

[7] Blouhos K, Boulas KA, Salpigktidis II, Konstantinidou A, Ioannidis K, Hatzigeorgiadis A (2013) Total Reconstruction of the Afferent Loop for Treatment of Radiation-Induced Afferent Loop Obstruction with Segmental Involvement after Pancreaticoduodenectomy with Roux-en-Y Reconstruction. *Case Rep Oncol* 6:424-429.

[8] Sarli L, Iusco D, Violi V, Roncoroni L (2003) Enterolith ileus complicating afferent loop syndrome simulating acute pancreatitis. 88:129-132.

[9] De Martino C, Caiazzo P, Albano M, Pastore M, Tramutoli PR, Rocca R, Botte M, Sigillito A (2012) Acute afferent loop obstruction treated by endoscopic decompression. Case report and review of literature. *Ann Ital Chir* 83:555-558.

[10] Grisé K, McFadden D (2001) Anastomotic technique influences outcomes after partial gastrectomy for adenocarcinoma. *Am Surg* 67:948-950.

[11] Kim DJ, Lee JH, Kim W (2013) Afferent loop obstruction following laparoscopic distal gastrectomy with Billroth-II gastrojejunostomy. *J Korean Surg Soc* 84:281-286 .

[12] Aoki M, Saka M, Morita S, Fukagawa T, Katai H (2010) Afferent loop obstruction after distal gastrectomy with Roux-en-Y reconstruction. *World J Surg* 34:2389-2392.

[13] Pannala R, Brandabur JJ, Gan SI, Gluck M, Irani S, Patterson DJ, Ross AS, Dorer R, Traverso LW, Picozzi VJ, Kozarek RA (2011) Afferent limb syndrome and delayed GI problems after pancreatic

oduodenectomy for pancreatic cancer: single-center, 14-year experience. *Gastrointest* Endosc 74:295-302.
[14] Vettoretto N, Pettinato G, Romessis M, Bravo AF, Barozzi G, Giovanetti M (2006) Laparoscopy in afferent loop obstruction presenting as acute pancreatitis. *JSLS* 10:270-274.
[15] Rana SV, Bhardwaj SB (2008) Small intestinal bacterial overgrowth. *Scand J Gastroenterol* 43:1030-1037.
[16] Lee MC, Bui JT, Knuttinen MG, Gaba RC, Scott Helton W, Owens CA (2009) Enterolith causing afferent loop obstruction: a case report and literature review. *Cardiovasc Intervent Radiol* 32:1091-2096.
[17] Kwong WT, Fehmi SM, Lowy AM, Savides TJ (2014) Enteral stenting for gastric outlet obstruction and afferent limb syndrome following pancreaticoduodenectomy. *Ann Gastroenterol* 27:413-417.
[18] Sandrasegaran K, Maglinte DD (2005) Imaging of small bowel-related complications following major abdominal surgery. *Eur J Radiol* 53:374-386.
[19] Zissin R (2004) CT findings of afferent loop syndrome after a subtotal gastrectomy with Roux-en-Y reconstruction. *Emerg Radiol* 10:201-203.
[20] Juan YH, Yu CY, Hsu HH, Huang GS, Chan DC, Liu CH, Tung HJ, Chang WC (2011) Using multidetector-row CT for the diagnosis of afferent loop syndrome following gastroenterostomy reconstruction. Yonsei Med J 52:574-580.
[21] Zissin R, Osadchy A, Gayer G (2007) Abdominal CT findings of delayed postoperative complications. *Can Assoc Radiol J* 58:200-211..
[22] Kim HC, Han JK, Kim KW, Kim YH, Yang HK, Kim SH, Won HJ, Lee KH, Choi BI (2003) Afferent loop obstruction after gastric cancer surgery: helical CT findings. *Abdom Imaging* 28:624-630.
[23] Czakó L, Takács T, Morvay Z, Csernay L, Lonovics J (2004) Diagnostic role of secretin-enhanced MRCP in patients with unsuccessful ERCP. *World J Gastroenterol* 10:3034-3038.
[24] Lomanto D, Pavone P, Laghi A, Panebianco V, Mazzocchi P, Fiocca F, Lezoche E, Passariello R, Speranza V (1997) Magnetic resonance-cholangiopancreatography in the diagnosis of biliopancreatic diseases. *Am J Surg* 174:33-38.
[25] Demirjian AN, Kent TS, Callery MP, Vollmer CM (2010) The inconsistent nature of symptomatic pancreatico-jejunostomy anastomotic strictures. *HPB* 12:482-487.

[26] Kim HJ, Park JY, Bang S, Park SW, Lee YC, Song SY (2009) Self-expandable metal stents for recurrent malignant obstruction after gastric surgery. *Hepatogastroenterology* 56:914-917.

[27] Hintze RE, Adler A, Veltzke W, Abou-Rebyeh H (1997) Endoscopic access to the papilla of Vater for endoscopic retrograde cholangiopancreatography in patients with billroth II or Roux-en-Y gastrojejunostomy. *Endoscopy*29:69-73.

[28] Sasaki T, Isayama H, Kogure H, Yamada A, Aoki T, Kokudo N, Koike K (2014) Double-balloon enteroscope-assisted enteral stent placement for malignant afferent-loop obstruction after Roux-en-Y reconstruction. *Endoscopy* 2014;46:541-542.

[29] Laasch HU (2010) Obstructive jaundice after bilioenteric anastomosis: transhepatic and direct percutaneous enteral stent insertion for afferent loop occlusion. *Gut Liver* 4:89-95.

[30] Reddy JR, Saxena R, Singh RK, Pottakkat B, Prakash A, Behari A, Gupta K, Kapoor VK (2012) Reoperation following Pancreaticoduodenectomy. *Int J Surg Oncol* 2012:218248.

[31] Blouhos K, Boulas KA, Tsiomita E, Papageorgiou I, Ioannidis K, Hatzigeorgiadis A (2014) Pancreaticojejuno-jejunostomy during reconstruction of the afferent loop in surgery of radiation-induced afferent loop obstruction following pancreaticoduodenectomy with Roux-en-Y reconstruction. *Updates Surg* 66:51-57 .

[32] Morgan KA, Fontenot BB, Harvey NR, Adams DB (2010) Revision of anastomotic stenosis after pancreatic head resection for chronic pancreatitis: is it futile? *HPB* 12:211-216.

[33] Chapter reviewed by Botsios D. MD, PhD, Professor of Surgery, Medical School, Aristotle University of Thessaloniki, Thessaloniki, Greece .

Reviewed by Botsios D. MD, PhD, Professor of Surgery, Medical School, Aristotle University of Thessaloniki, Thessaloniki, Greece

In: Intussusception and Bowel Obstruction
Editor: Rosie Miller
ISBN: 978-1-63482-703-4

Chapter 7

Decreasing Post-Surgical Adhesions That Cause Recurrent Small Bowel Obstructions with a Conservative Manual Physical Therapy

Amanda D. Rice,* [*] *PhD, and C. Richard King, III, MD
Clear Passage Physical Therapy, Gainesville, Florida, US

Abstract

Small bowel obstruction (SBO) is a common complication typically caused by adhesions that form after abdominal surgery, in response to inflammation associated with post-surgical healing. Adhesion formation occurs in an estimated 50-100% of abdominal or pelvic surgery patients and is the most common etiology of SBO. In the United States, adhesion-related SBO is a major health care expenditure annually.

Treatment options for adhesive SBO range from supportive care, consisting of bowel rest and intravenous fluids, to surgical intervention. While the non-invasive treatment options are effective at treating the

[*] Correspondence: Amanda D. Rice, Clear Passage Physical Therapy, 4421 NW 39th Ave Gainesville FL, 32606 USA. Tel. (352) 336-1433 Fax: (352) 336-9980 Email: amandar@clearpassage.com.

current obstructive episode, the underlying cause of the obstructions – adhesions -- is not addressed. Surgical intervention is effective in treating the adhesions causing the current obstruction; however, surgery is the primary cause of adhesion formation and, thus, patients with a history of adhesion formation are at risk for developing additional adhesions and subsequent obstructions requiring additional surgeries. There continues to be research -- with limited success -- into methods of adhesion formation reduction in surgical techniques, medications and adhesion barriers.

Manual physical therapy has been demonstrated to deform adhesions within the abdomen and pelvis, allowing the pelvic and abdominal tissues and to function more normally. The manipulation of soft tissues to generate systemic functional benefits is not a new concept. In the field of osteopathic manual therapy, skilled manipulation of the soft tissues has long been believed to affect biomechanical change in adhesions such that the involved tissues exhibit increased pliability and independence of mobility. We have demonstrated a high rate of success treating post-surgical adhesions that cause recurrent obstructions. Patients report long term benefits from treatment and improvements in overall quality of life. Treatment with manual physical therapy compared to standard treatments will be discussed in the context of recurrent small bowel obstructions.

Introduction

Small bowel obstruction (SBO) is a common life-threatening complication of surgery or abdominal trauma, typically caused by adhesions that form as a normal part of the healing process. When healing from surgery or any other injury or infection occurs, an inflammatory response is initiated to recruit the cells necessary to close the surgical incision and repair the tissues. As a side effect of this inflammatory response, adhesions form in tissues at and near the surgical repair or trauma site due to the presence of collagen and scar tissue mediators. There is a large variation in not only the presentation of the adhesions- thin and filmy to vascular and innervated thick tissue- but in the predictability of severity of adhesion formation. Surgical technique and experience, exposure to dry heat, degree of organ manipulation, inherent patient inflammation, post surgical infection and lysis of preexisting adhesions have all been implicated in post surgical adhesion formation [1–6]. With no definitive molecular target for prevention of adhesion formation the development of adhesion barriers or surgical additives to prevent adhesion formation has proven to be unsuccessful thus far [7–13].

Current estimations of 50-100% of surgical patients develop adhesions after abdominal or pelvic surgery [8, 14–18]. Adhesions have been implicated in chronic pain, infertility, bowel obstruction and general dysfunction, with symptoms appearing hours to years after the initiating insult or surgery. It has been estimated that up to 30% of surgical small bowel resection patients will undergo additional surgery due to adhesions within a 10 year period based upon large studies [19]. Rates of additional surgery for chronic pelvic pain in women are similar, with most benefits of pain reduction being maintained only 12 months.

The treatment guidelines for partial ASBO in the absence of bowel strangulation and peritonitis is supportive care to control the clinical symptoms to allow resolution of the obstruction without further intervention [20]. While this method of treatment is often effective in treating the current obstruction, this approach does not address the adhesions that are the primary cause of the obstruction or the risk of subsequent bowel obstructions. The only treatment currently available to treat adhesive bowel obstructions is surgery; this frequently causes the formation of additional adhesions. It has been suggested in the literature that once a patient enters the cycle of adhesion formation each subsequent surgery exponentially enhances the formation of additional adhesions. The risk of surgically induced bowel perforation increases with the presence of adhesions, increasing surgical risk to the patient in addition to increasing surgical time and effort.

The number of surgeries for adhesion related disease in 2010 was a staggering 381,364 in the US with an additional 100,335 patients undergoing bowel resection and an average 30 day readmission rate of 11-15% [21]. Thus, adhesion related disease causes significant surgical efforts, hospital resources and comprise major expenditures each year. Additionally, there is a considerable negative impact on the patients' quality of life from frequent hospital readmissions. Beyond the surgical risk and management of patients during an SBO episode, these patients experience a negative impact on their quality of life (QOL). The most commonly impacted area of life in these patients is diet, in which patients often follow a limited diet due to the risk of causing another bowel obstruction, leading often to serious health consequences from malnutrition.

A conservative therapy that decreases the risk of bowel obstruction in the absence of surgery is of significant importance to both patients and physicians. The approach to treating patients with recurrent adhesive SBOs discussed is a multifaceted approach in both treatment and outcome monitoring, with a focus on methods that are the least invasive possible.

The Clear Passage Approach

The Clear Passage Approach (CPA) is a manual physical therapy (mPT) protocol focused on the deformation of adhesions throughout the abdomen and pelvis. Historically mPT used to treat adults with a wide variety of adhesive conditions including burns, adhesive capsulitis, radiculopathy, pain, infertility and lessening of scars [22–31] and has shown promise in preventing adhesion formation in animal models [32,33]. The CPA hypothesized to deform the adhesions that cause SBO episodes, incorporating a variety of recognized manual soft tissue techniques, including myofascial release [34], osseous and visceral manipulation [35], craniosacral and other manual therapies, along with refinements and modifications of these techniques to treat patients in a patient-centered model [36]. Adhesion deformation is achieved by direct force applied in a site specific manner after identification of areas of tissue with decreased mobility. Tissue mobility is addressed in a systematic manner beginning with the most superficial structures followed by deeper structures and viscera. The amount and duration of force that is applied to cause these microfailures varies within the tolerance of each patient and according to the site of the body that is being treated. For example, the same technique applied to large muscle groups will use much greater force than that which is applied to more delicate areas, such as structures at the cranium, or abdominopelvic viscera.

The treatment is typically performed for four hours a day over five consecutive days with 20 hours being the standard treatment regimen for the CPA. Side effects from treatment are minimal and transient (often resolving before treatment hour 12, data not shown) as described in Table 1 with the most common being pain in the hip or back areas and abdominal tenderness. Given the treatment regimen and the level of manual pressures, these reported side effects are not unexpected and are mild when compared to the risks and side effects from surgical intervention.

Several case reports have been published describing the successful treatment and outcomes of patients with recurrent SBOs due to adhesions treated with the CPA. The first was a multiple case series published in the Journal of Clinical Medicine that included two adults with extensive abdominal and pelvic surgeries experiencing recurrent SBOs due to adhesions that were treated with the CPA with a focus on deformation of pelvic and abdominal adhesions [37]. Both patients had resolution of SBO symptoms and improvement in general health at the time of publication of the study.

Table 1. Summary of reported side effects from CPA treatment over the course of treatment by SBO patients. Reported side effects were assessed daily with conditions present before treatment subtracted to assess the rate of new side effects. n = 31.

Side Effect	Rate of Observation
Abdominal tenderness	19.4%
Fatigue	9.7%
Headache	12.9%
Pelvic or abdominal cramping	9.7%
Poor sleep	3.2%
Aching	32.3%
Bloating	3.2%
Nausea	12.9%
Diarrhea	12.9%
Emotional lability or irritability	9.7%
Vaginal spotting	5.0%
Skin tear	6.5%
Tailbone pain	9.7%
Hip or back pain	22.6%

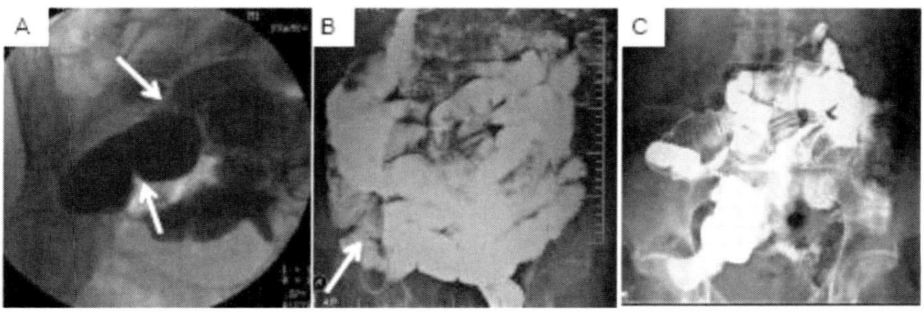

Figure 1. Small bowel radiographs of Patient 1 documenting SBO resolution over time. Arrows note areas of obstruction. (A) Before therapy in 2011: incomplete SBO due to adhesions visualized by X-ray showing dilation of the proximal mid ileum. (B) Twelve months after therapy in 2012: mild stricture at the terminal ileum with no other small bowel abnormalities. (C) After 40 h of therapy: normal small bowel series X-ray in 2012. Reprinted from J. Clin. Med. 2013, 2, 1-12; under a Creative Commons Attribution 4.0 International license.

Additional follow up with the patients has demonstrated long term benefits from the CPA treatment, with neither patient experiencing additional SBO episodes for 3 years. Figure 1 shows the timeline of small bowel X-rays throughout the course of treatment of the patient, demonstrating the resolution of adhesions and stricture that were present before CPA treatment.

A second case report, published in Pediatric Reports, described the treatment of a young child with extensive surgical history secondary to an open book pelvic fracture obtained in a motor vehicle accident. The accident trauma, 19 required surgeries, extended use of VAC dressing, and subsequent healing caused dense adhesion formation throughout his abdomen and pelvis. The adhesions caused pain, recurrent SBOs and one testicle to ascend into the pelvis. The child was treated using the CPA and reported decreased pain, absence of SBOs, an improved diet and the avoidance of another surgery as the ascending testicle returned to normal position.

The longevity of benefits from the CPA treatment has been assessed in multiple patient populations including patients with recurrent SBOs. In long term follow up with 31 patients (mean 19 months post treatment; range 11 months to 35 months post treatment) demonstrated positive outcomes that were maintained long term with lower than would be expected for long term readmissions of 30% (Table 2). The demonstration in this limited number of patients is encouraging and warrants further investigation as a treatment option for this patient population. The single surgery required post CPA treatment was for radiation enteritis, which CPA treatment is not theorized to treat based upon the disease process associated with those sections of bowel. Anecdotal information from this patient population suggests that 20 hours of treatment is adequate to eliminate or decrease the frequency SBO episodes, however, some patients may require additional treatment for complete resolution of symptoms. This is currently under investigation to determine predictors for patient populations that would benefit from additional treatment.

The preliminary data on the treatment of patients with recurrent SBO due to adhesions was encouraging and supported further investigation in prospective clinical trials. However, before any prospective trials could be undertaken a tool for measurement of outcomes specific to this patient population had to be developed. A validated questionnaire was developed at Clear Passage to specifically monitor changes and outcomes for treatments focused on patients with adhesive SBO. This SBO questionnaire (SBO-Q) assess the impact on the QOL of SBO patients across six domains including diet, gastrointestinal symptoms, pain, pain severity, overall quality of life and the requirement for medication [38]. In the validation study patients with a history of SBO reported negatively impacts in all measured domains as compared to a population of patients with no history of SBO or abdominal surgery.

Table 2. Rates of SBO and surgical intervention of patients after CPA treatment as compared to rates expected based upon the literature at a mean time of follow up of 19 months. P-values from odds ratio calculation using standard methods n = 31.

	CPA treated rate	Expected rate	P-value
Hospital admissions for SBO post treatment	7	9.3	0.5264
Surgery post treatment	1	9.3	0.0215

Therefore, improvements in quality of life and the return to a level comparable to patients with a low risk of adhesions is significant, particularly to the personal experiences and improvements to the individual patient's QOL.

Prospective clinical studies utilizing the SBO-Q for outcome measurements are currently underway for determining the efficacy of the CPA in treatment of adhesive SBO.

Conclusion

Observational care and bowel rest are preferred in non-emergency cases of SBO, supporting the desire to use the least invasive method to treat each subject. Therefore, a noninvasive technique to treat symptoms related to SBOs has precedent. The use of the CPA, a manual physical therapy protocol, to treat abdominal and pelvic adhesions causing SBOs and improve the QOL of patients has been shown to have positive long term effects on SBOs with no evidence of induction of adhesion formation that is observed with subsequent surgery [30]. The results from the case reports and long term follow up suggest that the CPA can be used to treat adhesions and scar adherence safely in the recurrent SBO subject population.

The CPA is effective at adhesion deformation measured by symptom resolution in both adult and pediatric populations. It has been noted in published studies, however, that pediatric patients are expected to require additional treatment with growth and physical development due to the impact on scar tissue present, as is documented in the literature in children with large dermatological grafts.

Large prospective studies will offer more power in determining efficacy rates and populations that benefit from the CPA treatment, providing guidance in surgical alternative for patients with adhesion related bowel obstructions.

References

[1] Brochhausen C, Schmitt VH, Planck CNE, Rajab TK, Hollemann D, Tapprich C, Krämer B, Wallwiener C, Hierlemann H, Zehbe R, Planck H, Kirkpatrick CJ. Current strategies and future perspectives for intraperitoneal adhesion prevention. *J. Gastrointest. Surg*. 2012;16(6):1256–74. doi:10.1007/s11605-011-1819-9.

[2] Hellebrekers BWJ, Kooistra T. Pathogenesis of postoperative adhesion formation. *Br. J. Surg*. 2011;98(11):1503–16. doi:10.1002/bjs.7657.

[3] Ouaïssi M, Gaujoux S, Veyrie N, Denève E, Brigand C, Castel B, Duron JJ, Rault a, Slim K, Nocca D. Post-operative adhesions after digestive surgery: their incidence and prevention: review of the literature. *J. Visc. Surg*. 2012;149(2):e104–14. doi:10.1016/j.jviscsurg.2011.11.006.

[4] Attard J-AP, MacLean AR. Adhesive small bowel obstruction: epidemiology, biology and prevention. *Can J Surg*. 2007;50(4):291–300. Available at: http://www.pubmedcentral.nih. gov/articlerender. fcgi? artid=2386166&tool=pmcentrez&rendertype=abstract.

[5] Barmparas G, Branco BC, Schnüriger B, Lam L, Inaba K, Demetriades D. The incidence and risk factors of post-laparotomy adhesive small bowel obstruction. *J. Gastrointest. Surg*. 2010;14(10):1619–28. doi:10. 1007/s11605-010-1189-8.

[6] Ten Broek RPG, Issa Y, van Santbrink EJP, Bouvy ND, Kruitwagen RFPM, Jeekel J, Bakkum EA, Rovers MM, van Goor H. Burden of adhesions in abdominal and pelvic surgery: systematic review and met-analysis. *BMJ*. 2013;347:f5588. Available at: http://www.ncbi.nlm.nih. gov/pmc/articles/PMC3789584/pdf/bmj.f5588.pdf. Accessed October 9, 2013.

[7] Pismensky S V, Kalzhanov ZR, Eliseeva MY, Kosmas IP, Mynbaev O a. Severe inflammatory reaction induced by peritoneal trauma is the key driving mechanism of postoperative adhesion formation. *BMC Surg*. 2011;11(1):30. doi:10.1186/1471-2482-11-30.

[8] Arung W, Meurisse M, Detry O. Pathophysiology and prevention of postoperative peritoneal adhesions. *World J. Gastroenterol*. 2011;17(41):4545–53. doi:10.3748/wjg.v17.i41.4545.

[9] Yigitler C, Karakas IDO, Kucukodacı IIZ, Cosar IIIA, Bu I V. Adhesion-preventing properties of 4% icodextrin and canola oil : a comparative experimental study. 2012;67(11):1303–1308. doi:10.6061/clinics/2012(11)14.
[10] Cheong YC, Shelton JB, Laird SM, Richmond M, Kudesia G, Li TC, Ledger WL. IL-1, IL-6 and TNF-alpha concentrations in the peritoneal fluid of women with pelvic adhesions. *Hum. Reprod.* 2002;17(1):69–75. Available at: http://humrep.oxfordjournals.org/content/17/1/69.long.
[11] Ten Broek RPG, Wilbers J, van Goor H. Electrocautery causes more ischemic peritoneal tissue damage than ultrasonic dissection. *Surg Endosc.* 2011;25(6):1827–34. doi:10.1007/s00464-010-1474-3.
[12] Cahill RA, Redmond HP. Cytokine orchestration in post-operative peritoneal adhesion formation. *World J. Gastroenterol.* 2008;14 (31):4861–6. Available at: http://www.ncbi.nlm.nih.gov/pmc/ articles /PMC2739937/pdf/WJG-14-4861.pdf. Accessed July 29, 2014.
[13] Lauder CIW, Garcea G, Strickland A, Maddern GJ. Abdominal adhesion prevention: still a sticky subject? *Dig. Surg.* 2010;27(5):347–58. doi:10.1159/000314805.
[14] Menzies D, Ellis H. Intestinal obstruction from adhesions--how big is the problem? *Ann. R. Coll. Surg. Engl.* 1990;72(1):60–3. Available at: http://www.ncbi.nlm.nih.gov/pmc/articles/PMC2499092/. Accessed September 5, 2012.
[15] diZerega GS. Contemporary adhesion prevention. *Fertil Steril.* 1994;61(2):219–35. Available at: http://www.ncbi.nlm.nih.gov/pubmed/ 8299773. Accessed September 5, 2012.
[16] Kössi J, Salminen P, Rantala A, Laato M. Population-based study of the surgical workload and economic impact of bowel obstruction caused by postoperative adhesions. *Br. J. Surg.* 2003;90(11):1441–4. doi:10.1002/ bjs.4272.
[17] Brüggmann D, Tchartchian G, Wallwiener M, Münstedt K, Tinneberg H-R, Hackethal A. Intra-abdominal adhesions: definition, origin, significance in surgical practice, and treatment options. *Dtsch. Arztebl. Int.* 2010;107(44):769–75. doi:10.3238/arztebl.2010.0769.
[18] Di Saverio S, Coccolini F, Galati M, Smerieri N, Biffl WL, Ansaloni L, Tugnoli G, Velmahos GC, Sartelli M, Bendinelli C, Fraga GP, Kelly MD, Moore F a, Mandalà V, Mandalà S, Masetti M, Jovine E, Pinna AD, Peitzman AB, Leppaniemi A, Sugarbaker PH, Goor H Van, Moore EE, Jeekel J, Catena F. Bologna guidelines for diagnosis and management of adhesive small bowel obstruction (ASBO): 2013 update

of the evidence-based guidelines from the world society of emergency surgery ASBO working group. *World J. Emerg. Surg*. 2013;8(1):42. doi:10.1186/1749-7922-8-42.

[19] Wilson MS, Ellis H, Menzies D, Moran BJ, Parker MC, Thompson JN. A review of the management of small bowel obstruction. Members of the Surgical and Clinical Adhesions Research Study (SCAR). *Ann. R. Coll. Surg. Engl*. 1999;81(5):320–8. Available at: http://www.ncbi.nlm.nih.gov/pmc/articles/PMC2503289/. Accessed September 5, 2012.

[20] Di Saverio S, Coccolini F, Galati M, Smerieri N, Biffl WL, Ansaloni L, Tugnoli G, Velmahos GC, Sartelli M, Bendinelli C, Fraga GP, Kelly MD, Moore FA, Mandalà V, Mandalà S, Masetti M, Jovine E, Pinna AD, Peitzman AB, Leppaniemi A, Sugarbaker PH, Goor H Van, Moore EE, Jeekel J, Catena F, Van Goor H. Bologna guidelines for diagnosis and management of adhesive small bowel obstruction (ASBO): 2013 update of the evidence-based guidelines from the world society of emergency surgery ASBO working group. *World J. Emerg. Surg*. 2013;8(1):42. doi:10.1186/1749-7922-8-42.

[21] HCUPnet: A tool for identifying, tracking, and analyzing national hospital statistics. 2012. Available at: http://hcupnet.ahrq.gov/HCUPnet.jsp?Id=6D36343307A90AD9&Form=SelLAY&JS=Y&Action=>>Next>>&_LAY=Researcher. Accessed October 8, 2012.

[22] Sucher BM. Ultrasonography-Guided Osteopathic Manipulative Treatment for a Patient With Thoracic Outlet Syndrome. *J. Am. Osteopat. Assoc*. 2011;111(9):543–547. Available at: http://www.jaoa.org/content/ 111/9/543.long. Accessed November 5, 2012.

[23] Sampson S, Meng M, Schulte A, Trainor D, Montenegro R, Aufiero D. Management of Dupuytren contracture with ultrasound-guided lidocaine injection and needle aponeurotomy coupled with osteopathic manipulative treatment. *J. Am. Osteopat. Assoc*. 2011;111(2):113–6. Available at: http://www.jaoa.org/content/111/2/113.long.

[24] Boyles R, Toy P, Mellon J, Hayes M, Hammer B. Effectiveness of manual physical therapy in the treatment of cervical radiculopathy: a systematic review. *J Man Manip Ther*. 2011;19(3):135–42. doi:10.1179/2042618611Y.0000000011.

[25] Bayliss AJ, Klene FJ, Gundeck EL, Loghmani MT. Treatment of a patient with post-natal chronic calf pain utilizing instrument-assisted soft tissue mobilization: a case study. *J. Man Manip. Ther*. 2011;19(3):127–34. doi:10.1179/2042618611Y.0000000006.

[26] Şenbursa G, Baltaci G, Atay ÖA. The effectiveness of manual therapy in supraspinatus tendinopathy. *Acta Orthop. Traumatol.* 2011;45(3):162–7. Available at: http://www.aott.org.tr/article/view/5000011471/5000011840. Accessed November 5, 2012.

[27] Gaspar PD, Willis FB. Adhesive capsulitis and dynamic splinting: a controlled, cohort study. *BMC Musculoskelet Disord.* 2009;10:111. doi:10.1186/1471-2474-10-111.

[28] Wurn LJ, Wurn BF, King CR, Roscow AS, Scharf ES, Shuster JJ. Increasing orgasm and decreasing dyspareunia by a manual physical therapy technique. *MedGenMed.* 2004;6(4):47. Available at: http://www.ncbi.nlm.nih.gov/pmc/articles/PMC1480593/. Accessed September 4, 2012.

[29] Wurn BF, Wurn LJ, Patterson K, King CR, Scharf ES. Decreasing dyspareunia and dysmenorrhea in women with endometriosis via a manual physical therapy: Results from two independent studies. *J. Endometr.* 2011;3(4):188–196. doi:10.5301/JE.2012.9088.

[30] Wurn BF, Wurn LJ, King CR, Heuer M a, Roscow AS, Hornberger K, Scharf ES. Treating fallopian tube occlusion with a manual pelvic physical therapy. *Altern. Ther. Heal. Med.* 2008;14(1):18–23. Available at: http://www.ncbi.nlm.nih.gov/pubmed/18251317.

[31] Wurn BF, Wurn LJ, King CR, Heuer MA, Roscow AS, Scharf ES, Shuster JJ. Treating female infertility and improving IVF pregnancy rates with a manual physical therapy technique. *MedGenMed.* 2004;6(2):51. Available at: http://www.ncbi.nlm.nih.gov/pmc/ articles/PMC1395760/. Accessed September 4, 2012.

[32] Bove GM, Chapelle SL. Visceral mobilization can lyse and prevent peritoneal adhesions in a rat model. *J. Bodyw. Mov. Ther.* 2012;16(1):76–82. doi:10.1016/j.jbmt.2011.02.004.

[33] Chapelle SL, Bove GM. Visceral massage reduces postoperative ileus in a rat model. *J. Bodyw. Mov. Ther.* 2013;17(1):83–8. doi:10.1016/j.jbmt.2012.05.004.

[34] Cantu RI, Grodin AJ. *Myofascial Manipulation: Theory and Clinical Application.* Gaithersburg: Aspen Publishers; 1992:77–78, 86–88.

[35] Langenau EE, Dowling DJ, Dyer C, Roberts WL. Frequency of specific osteopathic manipulative treatment modalities used by candidates while taking COMLEX-USA Level 2-PE. *J. Am. Osteopath. Assoc.* 2012;112(8):509–13. Available at: http://www.jaoa.org/content/112/8/509.long. Accessed September 16, 2013.

[36] Miles A. Science, humanism, judgement, ethics: person-centered medicine as an emergent model of modern clinical practice. *Folia Med (Plovdiv)*. 2013;55(1):5–24. Available at: http://www.ncbi.nlm.nih.gov/pubmed/23905483. Accessed September 19, 2013.

[37] Rice A, King R, Reed E, Patterson K, Wurn B, Wurn L. Manual Physical Therapy for Non-Surgical Treatment of Adhesion-Related Small Bowel Obstructions: Two Case Reports. *J. Clin. Med.* 2013;2(1):1–12. doi:10.3390/jcm2010001.

[38] Rice AD, Wakefield LB, Patterson K, Reed ED, Wurn BF, Klingenberg B, King CR, Wurn LJ. Development and validation of a questionnaire to measure serious and common quality of life issues for patients experiencing small bowel obstructions. *Healthcare*. 2014;2(1):139–149. doi:10.3390/healthcare2010139.

In: Intussusception and Bowel Obstruction
Editor: Rosie Miller
ISBN: 978-1-63482-703-4

Chapter 8

Alternative Treatment of Non-Malignant Bowel Obstruction in Patients with Gynecological Cancer

C. Richard King, III, MD,* and Amanda D. Rice, PhD
Clear Passage Physical Therapy, Gainesville, Florida, US

Abstract

Bowel obstructions in patients with primary or metastasized cancer within the abdomen and pelvis are common occurrences. These patients experience bowel obstructions due to two distinct etiologies, malignant or non-malignant. The malignant cause of bowel obstruction is a mass obstructing the bowel, while non-malignant obstructions are the result of adhesions disrupting normal bowel function. Adhesion formation in response to radiation, chemotherapy, surgery and other treatments for the malignancy occur in 50-100% of gynecological cancer patients.

Treatment options for bowel obstruction are limited regardless of etiology. Patients undergoing treatment for cancer or that are considered palliative are often not surgical candidates and treatment is supportive

* Corresponding author: C. Richard King, III, Clear Passage Physical Therapy, 4421 NW 39th Ave Gainesville FL, 32606 US. Tel: (352) 336-1433, fax: (352) 336-9980, e-mail: richardk @clearpassage.com.

with the goal of decreasing symptoms and pain control. Supportive care is often effective in resolving the current obstruction; but, patients are often on restricted diets and experience a significantly decreased quality of life due to recurrent partial or total bowel obstructions.

There is a significant interest in non-invasive treatment options that improve quality of life for these patients. We have demonstrated efficacy of a manual physical therapy regimen in treating non-malignant bowel obstructions in both active cancer patients as well as those who are in remission and are experiencing bowel obstructions due to surgery and treatment of the malignancy. A literature review of traditional medical treatment options and our experience in treating gynecological cancer patients with non-malignant bowel obstruction using manual physical therapy is presented.

Introduction

Gynecologic carcinoma, including cervical, vaginal, ovarian and uterine cancer, is the fourth leading cause of cancer related deaths in women. One complication of the treatment of these cancers is bowel obstruction, with estimates of up to 35% of all women with gynecologic cancer experiencing bowel obstructions [1–8]. Bowel obstructions for these patients classifiedas either of two etiologies, malignant or non-malignant with development of the obstructions being generally a gradual process rather than a sudden acute event [1, 2, 9]. The malignant cause of bowel obstruction is from a mass obstructing the bowel, while the non-malignant obstructions are the result of adhesions disrupting normal bowel function. This chapter will focus on the treatment options for patients with adhesive type bowel obstructions.

Cancer growth, particularly solid tumors, are known to induce inflammation for sustained growth and enhancement of angiogenesis [10, 11]. Standard treatment for gynecological cancer includes surgical hysterectomy, oophrectomy and excision of affected tissues in the pelvis in concert with radiation and chemotherapy. All of these treatments have been documented to induce inflammation as a part of the healing process [12, 13]. Inflammation is the driving force of adhesion formation with surgery identified as a leading cause of abdominal and pelvic adhesion formation [14–20], therefore it is not surprising that a large number of patients experience bowel obstruction due to adhesions. Depending on the severity of the obstruction, prognosis and wishes of the patient, traditional intervention options of a bowel obstruction vary from management with medications, nasogastric tube, percutaenous gastrostomy, placement of a bowel stent and/or surgical intervention including adhesiolysis and bowel resection [1, 21–23].

It has been reported that women with gynecological cancer who undergo surgery for bowel obstruction have a survival time of less than 12 months due to complications from the SBO, surgical interventions for the SBO, and other comorbidities [5, 24]. This increased risk makes treatment recommendations while attempting to maintain quality of life for these patients is challenging. The use of surgery for palliative treatment of SBO secondary to ovarian cancer has been demonstrated to be associated with high morbidity and mortality, with mortality rates of 13-22%, particularly in patients with advanced disease [1, 6–8, 25]. Many cancer patients use alternative medicine during the course of their treatment and for side effects of the disease, particularly pain and constipation [26–35]. Often, these patients are not surgical candidates at the end of the disease progression and abdominal massage has been show to be beneficial in symptom management and improvement in quality of life [21, 29, 31, 33, 34].

Patients that have undergone treatment for gynecological cancer also experience SBOs due to adhesions, sometimes decades after their treatment for cancer. The treatment options for these patients is limited with recurrent SBO episodes being commonly experienced. In the absence of bowel strangulation and peritonitis, the current recommendations to manage adhesive small bowel obstructions apply diagnostic imaging, clinical symptomology and supportive care for the first 72 hours to allow the blockage adequate time to resolve independent of surgery [36]. While sometimes effective in treating the current obstruction, this approach does not address the internal adhesions or the risk of subsequent bowel obstructions. The only treatment currently available to treat adhesive bowel obstructions is surgery, which frequently causes new adhesions.

A number of surgical techniques, modifications, and adhesion preventing medications and barriers have been investigated, but no solution has been shown to completely prevent the formation of adhesions to date [13, 37–42]. Thus, any conservative therapy that decreases the risk of bowel obstruction in the absence of surgery is of significant importance.

Recently a manual physical therapy treatment for adhesive related disease has been shown to decrease adhesive bowel obstruction in both palliative and routine patients with a history of gynecological cancer.

Manual Physical Therapy Treatment

The alternative treatment is an intensive manual physical therapy termed the Clear Passage Approach (CPA) that utilizes methods and modifications of standard physical therapy modalities including myofascial release, muscle energy, craniosacral therapy, strain-counterstrain, Wurn Technique, and visceral manipulation. The manual physical therapy protocols utilized by the therapists have been previously described in other studies where the primary focus of therapy was the decrease of adhesions, and the outcomes were a return of normal mobility and motility to previously adhered organs [43–50].

The treatment focuses around the manual deformation of the adhesions using direct force in which the therapists identified areas of restricted mobility or motility of the organs and tissues. The amount and duration of force that is applied to cause microfailures of the adhesions causing obstructions and dysfunction can be significant, but varies within the tolerance of each patient and according to the site of the body that is being treated. The manual physical therapy approach is a combination of site-specific manipulation at adhered viscera combined with a whole body treatment, treating not only the abdomen in these patients, but also other areas of the body in which decreased function or mobility was identified during the initial evaluation. The therapists assessed tissue temperature, moisture, shear, extensibility and texture throughout the abdominopelvic viscera, with a special focus on areas deep to surgical scars. Testing visceral mobility consisted of the therapist palpating the tissues, then making precise manual movements to assess the ability of the organs to move directly over surrounding organs and tissues. In previously published trials and studies, these techniques increased mobility and decreased pain in patients with significant surgical histories that indicate adhesion formation [45, 48–51].

Palliative Case Series

Between the years of 2010 and 2012, six palliative care patients diagnosed with gynecological cancer and exhibiting present or recurrent small bowel obstructions due to abdominal and pelvic adhesions, were treated via the CPA. The average age of these patients was 55.3 years. All had previously undergone chemotherapy treatment for cancer and 4/6 had undergone radiation treatment for the current cancer (Table 1). The patients were treated in one-hour increments, with 5/6 of the patients undergoing treatment 4 hours a day for consecutive days due to not residing local to the physical therapy clinic. One patient was local to the clinic and attended treatment for 1-2 hours a week for 2 months. Approximately 85% of the manual physical therapy treatment time was focused directly on the adhered areas of the abdomen and pelvis for the patients presented in this case report.

Table 1. Demographics of palliative patients

Patient	Age at Treatment	Race	Education Level	Number of Hours Treated	Number of Days Treated	Type of cancer	Chemotherapy	Radiation	Pelvic Adhesions[1]	Number of SBO episodes before CPA	TPN/IV use at Treatment
1	49	Native American	2 years college	20	5	Ovarian	Y	Y	Y	1[2]	-
2	53	Caucasian	4 years college	16	4	Ovarian	Y	Y	Y	8[2]	Y
3	55	Caucasian	Unknown	16	4	Cervical	Y	Y	-	4[2]	Y
4	61	Caucasian	High school	13	60	Ovarian	Y	-	Y	3	-
5	57	Caucasian	2 years college	20	5	Cervical	Y	Y	Y	2	-
6	57	Caucasian	Unknown	28	9	Ovarian/ endometrial	Y	Y	Y	2	-

[1]Medical diagnosis of adhesions present. - = absent, Y = present.
[2]Patient was currently experiencing a partial or full bowel obstruction at the time of treatment.

The remainder of the time was spent treating other areas of the body causing pain and dysfunction, and instructing patients in home exercises and a home maintenance program. While all were palliative care patients experiencing recurrent bowel obstructions or symptoms of nonmalignant bowel obstruction, it is important to note that only 3 of the 6 patients required TPN or IV and liquids only for nutrition at the time of treatment. Of the remaining three patients, 1 was on a liquid only diet while the remaining 2 patients had no dietary restrictions unless experiencing an active bowel obstruction episode. All patients were ambulatory at the time of treatment.

There was a large variation in past medical history and current pain reports (Table 2) for the patients, with abdominal pain being the only shared current pain complaint. Five of six patients had a history of previous abdominal and/or pelvic surgery, likely contributing to the presence of adhesive disease causing the recurrent bowel obstructions (Table 3).

The single patient with no history of abdominal/pelvic surgery did have a pelvic mass likely contributing to the recurrent bowel obstructions; however, it was assumed that she did have abdominal adhesions from radiation treatments and was not a surgical candidate for the pelvic mass at the time of treatment.

Table 2. Past medical history and current pain complaints for palliative patients

Patient	Bladder Infection	Sexual Dysfunction	Endometrosis	Infertility	Uterine Fibroids	Vaginal Infection	Constipation	Digestive Problems	Intestinal Problems	Gall Stones	Abdominal Pain	Pelvic Pain	Headache	Back Pain	Intercourse Pain	Neck Pain	Edema
1	-	-	-	Y	Y	-	Y	Y	Y	-	Y	-	-	-	Y	Y	Y
2	-	-	Y	-	-	-	Y	Y	Y	-	Y	-	-	-	-	-	-
3	-	Y	-	-	-	-	-	-	-	-	Y	Y	-	Y	-	-	Y
4	Y	Y	-	-	-	Y	Y	Y	Y	Y	Y	-	Y	-	Y	-	Y
5	-	Y	-	-	-	Y	Y	Y	Y	Y	Y	-	-	-	Y	-	Y
6	Y	Y	-	-	-	-	-	-	Y	-	Y	-	-	-	Y	-	-

(-) not present in medical history (Y) present in medical history.

Table 3. Total number of previous abdominal and pelvic surgeries for palliative patients

Patient	Abdominal/ Pelvic	Bowel Resection	Laparotomy	Laparoscopy	Hysterectomy	Omentectomy	Cholecystectomy
1	5	0	3	1	1	1	0
2	5	1	4	0	1	0	0
3	0	0	0	0	0	0	0
4	4	0	0	3	1	0	0
5	3	1	2	1	1	0	1
6	6	0	5	0	1	1	0

Two patients were unable to complete treatment (patients 2 and 3), undergoing only 16 hours of treatment, one due to a bladder infection and dehydration and the other due to progression of a bowel obstruction. Both were hospitalized prior to completion of treatment.

These patients required TPN nutrition at the initiation of treatment, had the most advanced cancer, and were physically the weakest at the time of treatment. Although these two patients did not complete treatment program, they did not experience any serious adverse reactions to treatment, and surgery was not required for the patient experiencing a bowel obstruction.

One patient with a history of edema did experience an increase in lower extremity and abdominal edema post treatment that resolved with use of compression garments (patient 5). The remaining three patients with a history of edema did not report an increase in edema post treatment (Table 1).

Survival time post treatment was not predictive of response to treatment nor was the ability to complete treatment predictive of survival time post treatment. All patients, including those who were unable to complete treatment, reported an improvement in their bowel obstruction symptoms and decrease frequency of obstruction symptoms post treatment. An improvement in overall pain levels were improved in 5/6 patients, with 6/6 patients demonstrating a decrease in bowel related pain. The patient that did not experience a decrease in overall pain had a solid mass tumor at the pancreas that was the cause of her residual pain (patient 6). Treatment was not anticipated to influence the pain experienced as a result of the tumor in that patient, however the SBO symptoms she experienced were improved.

Post Cancer Treatment Case Series

Post treatment gynecological patients considered cancer free but experiencing adhesive SBO were also treated via the CPA. The patients in this group were monitored for outcomes via the validated SBO Questionnaire (SBO-Q) that assesses the degree to which the patient's life is impacted with their SBO symptoms. This questionnaire assess five domains: diet, pain, gastrointestinal symptoms, medication requirements and overall quality of life; and the degree of pain is analyzed separately [52]. The SBO-Q was administered before CPA treatment and then 90 days after treatment. The questionnaire was scored and each patient assessed form improvement of quartiles based upon the criteria outlined in the SBO-Q validation study [52].

The average age of this group of six patients was 67.9 years. There were three patients that had undergone radiation treatment without chemotherapy, one that was treated with both chemotherapy and radiation; one patient that was treated with chemotherapy only and one patient that had no treatment beyond surgical intervention (Table 4).

Table 4. Demographics of post cancer treatment patients

Patient	Age at Treatment	Race	Education Level	Number of Hours Treated	Number of Days Treated	Type of cancer	Chemotherapy	Radiation	Pelvic Adhesions[1]	Number of SBO episodes before CPA
7	82	Caucasian	4 years college	40	10	Cervical	Y	Y	Y	9
8	88	Caucasian	6 years college	20	5	Endometrial	-	Y	Y	5
9	68	Caucasian	4 years college	20	5	Ovarian	Y	-	Y	3
10	65	Caucasian	Unknown	40	10	Cervical	-	Y	Y	21
11	54	Caucasian	4 years college	20	5	Endometrial	-	Y	Y	4
12	51	Caucasian	Unknown	20	5	Endometrial and Ovarian	-	-	Y	10

[1]Medical diagnosis of adhesions present. - = absent, Y= present.

All of the patients received intensive treatment of 4 hours a day with 4 or 6 patients undergoing treatment for 20 hours over 5 days, and 2 patients (numbers 7 and 10) receiving 40 hours over 2 weeks time. This patient population was stable; therefore, intensive treatment was tolerated well with no adverse events. The percent of manual therapy time focused on the abdomen and pelvis was similar to that of the palliative patient group.

The distribution of degree of impact for each of the domains in the SBO-Q was performed. Table 5 shows the total number of subjects in each domain by the SBO-Q established quartiles for classification of degree of impact on life, allowing for observation of clinically relevant trends.

Although no domains were significant by a T-test analysis, there was a clear trend of improvement in all domains, with more subjects classified as "normal" after treatment. There was significant improvement in reported pain ratings ($p = 0.00014$) and a general trend of improvement in the duration of time that the patient experienced pain (Table 6).

These observations were in line with patient reported subjective outcomes as well. The single patient that reported a negative change in respect to their diet was attributed to dietary restrictions related to prevention of bowel obstructions.

A larger study with long term follow up is underway with post cancer treatment patients with recurrent SBO.

Table 5. Distribution of patients for each of the domains in the SBO-Q for degree of impact quartiles. Patients completed the SBO-Q before treatment (pre treatment) and 90 days after completion of treatment (post treatment)

	Pre Treatment				Post Treatment				
	Normal	Minimum	Moderate	Severe	Normal	Minimum	Moderate	Severe	p-value
Diet	2	1	3	0	4	0	1	1	0.5761
Pain	3	2	1	0	6	0	0	0	0.1019
GI symptoms	2	4	0	0	6	0	0	0	0.0250
QOL	3	3	0	0	5	1	0	0	0.1747
Medication	4	0	1	1	5	0	1	0	0.5177

Quartiles were determined following the scoring criteria established during the validation of the SBO-Q. The number of patients in the quartiles for each domain assessed in the SBO-Q with pretreatment numbers compared to distribution post treatment. P-values for each domain via a 2-tailed paired T-test are given.

Table 6. Improvements in pain ratings and duration of pain. The average pain ratings using the standard 0 to 10 pain scale and pain duration as outlined in the SBO-Q before and after treatment are compared

	Pre-Treatment Average ± SD	Post Treatment Average ± SD	p-value
Maximum Pain Rating	7.7 ± 1.4	1.3 ± 1.4	0.00014
Pain Duration	4.3 ± 1.2	1.3 ± 1.0	0.01172

P-values for each domain via a 2-tailed paired T-test are given.

Conclusion

Manual physical therapy as a less invasive option to treat nonmalignant bowel obstruction in palliative patients is supported in the literature, in which surgery for palliation is controversial. Other studies have demonstrated improvement of QOL of patients experiencing pain and bowel obstruction symptoms near the end of life when physical therapy and abdominal massage were used [3, 21, 26, 29, 31–33, 43, 53]. Here we have described the treatment of 2 groups of six patients with either active or previous gynecological cancer experiencing bowel obstructions secondary to the presence of abdominal and pelvic adhesions via manual physical therapy. All patients experienced a decrease in pain associated with pelvic and abdominal adhesions, with the greatest improvements in the previous cancer treatment patients.

There were no adverse events reported following treatment of post-gynecological cancer treatment patients, with outcomes similar to those observed in post-surgical treatment patients.

Three palliative patients experienced adverse events during treatment, likely due to the extensiveness of their disease progression and physical condition at the time of treatment rather than directly related to treatment.

Based upon the data, it is suggestive that patients with recurring SBO with gynecological cancer may benefit from a protocol of manual physical therapy as described here. However, those with advanced disease, poor physical strength and relying upon IV or TPN for nutrition should be carefully screened for not only tolerance to treatment but also the effects of travel to the patient's ability to tolerate intensive treatment. Furthermore, patients with a history of edema formation should undergo further assessment prior to undergoing manual physical therapy by their physicians to ensure the procedures will not exacerbate the condition. Complications to all treatment options are to be expected in a palliative care population, particularly for a population experiencing recurrent bowel obstruction; however, it is important to consider patient goals for treatment and a realistic expectation of outcome when making recommendations. The patients presented in this case series had a realistic expectation of decreasing abdominal adhesions causing SBOs and SBO symptoms.Further studies are needed to identify predictors for treatment outcomes in a palliative care population and assess the long term effects and direct benefit of manual physical therapy to this patient population.

References

[1] Mangili, G., Aletti, G., Frigerio, L., Franchi, M., Panacci, N., Viganò, R., De Marzi, P., Zanetto, F., Ferrari, A. Palliative care for intestinal obstruction in recurrent ovarian cancer: a multivariate analysis. *Int. J. Gynecol. Cancer*. 2005;15(5):830–5. doi:10.1111/j.1525-1438.2005.00144.x.

[2] Bryan, D. N., Radbod, R., Berek, J. S. An analysis of surgical versus chemotherapeutic intervention for the management of intestinal obstruction in advanced ovarian cancer. *Int. J. Gynecol. Cancer*. 2006;16 (1):125–34. doi:10.1111/j.1525-1438.2006.00283.x.

[3] Barbera, L., Elit, L., Krzyzanowska, M., Saskin, R., Bierman, A. S. End of life care for women with gynecologic cancers. *Gynecol. Oncol*. 2010; 118(2):196–201. doi:10.1016/j.ygyno.2010.04.014.

[4] Herrinton, L. J., Neslund-Dudas, C., Rolnick, S. J., Hornbrook, M. C., Bachman, D. J., Darbinian, J. A., Jackson, J. M., Coughlin, S. S. Complications at the end of life in ovarian cancer. *J. Pain Symptom Manage*. 2007;34(3):237–43. doi:10.1016/j.jpainsymman.2006.11.011.

[5] Kolomainen, D. F., Barton, D. P. J. Surgical management of bowel obstruction in gynaecological malignancies. *Curr. Opin. Support Palliat. Care*. 2011;5(1):55–9. doi:10.1097/SPC.0b013e3283436d1b.

[6] Sartori, E., Chiudinelli, F., Pasinetti, B., Sostegni, B., Maggino, T. Possible role of palliative surgery for bowel obstruction in advanced ovarian cancer patients. *Eur. J. Gynaecol. Oncol*. 2010;31(1):31–6. Available at: http://www.ncbi.nlm.nih.gov/pubmed/20349778. Accessed April 12, 2013.

[7] Parveen, Z., Qureshi, A. N., Akbar, M., Zafar, A., Subhani, A. Palliative surgery for intestinal obstruction due to recurrent ovarian cancer. *J. Ayub. Med. Coll. Abbottabad*. 2009;21(1):135–136.

[8] Mooney, S. J., Winner, M., Hershman, D. L., Wright, J. D., Feingold, D. L., Allendorf, J. D., Neugut, A. I. Bowel obstruction in elderly ovarian cancer patients: A population-based study. *Gynecol. Oncol*. 2013;129(1): 107–12. doi:10.1016/j.ygyno.2012.12.028.

[9] Ripamonti, C., Bruera, E. Palliative management of malignant bowel obstruction. *Int. J. Gynecol. Cancer*. 2002;12(2):135–43. Available at: http://www.ncbi.nlm.nih.gov/pubmed/11975672.

[10] Mor, G., Yin, G., Chefetz, I., Yang, Y., Alvero, A. Ovarian cancer stem cells and inflammation. *Cancer Biol. Ther*. 2011;11(8):708–13. Available at: http://www.pubmedcentral.nih.gov/articlerender.fcgi?artid =3100563andtool=pmcentrezandrendertype=abstract.
Accessed February 26, 2015.

[11] Eskander, R. N., Tewari, K. S. Targeting angiogenesis in advanced cervical cancer. *Ther. Adv. Med. Oncol*. 2014;6(6):280–92. doi:10.1177/ 1758834014543794.

[12] Hellebrekers, B. W. J., Kooistra, T. Pathogenesis of postoperative adhesion formation. *Br. J. Surg*. 2011;98(11):1503–16. doi:10.1002/bjs.7657.

[13] Pismensky, S. V., Kalzhanov, Z. R., Eliseeva, M. Y., Kosmas, I. P., Mynbaev, O. A. Severe inflammatory reaction induced by peritoneal trauma is the key driving mechanism of postoperative adhesion formation. *BMC Surg*. 2011;11(1):30. doi:10.1186/1471-2482-11-30.

[14] Van Goor, H. Consequences and complications of peritoneal adhesions. *Colorectal Dis*. 2007;9 Suppl. 2:25–34. doi:10.1111/j.1463-1318.2007.01358.x.

[15] Coccolini, F., Ansaloni, L., Manfredi, R., Campanati, L., Poiasina, E., Bertoli, P., Capponi, M. G., Sartelli, M., Di Saverio, S., Cucchi, M., Lazzareschi, D., Pisano, M., Catena, F. Peritoneal adhesion index (PAI): proposal of a score for the "ignored iceberg" of medicine and surgery. *World J. Emerg. Surg*. 2013;8(1):6. doi:10.1186/1749-7922-8-6.

[16] Ouaïssi, M., Gaujoux, S., Veyrie, N., Denève, E., Brigand, C., Castel, B., Duron, J. J., Rault, A., Slim, K., Nocca, D. Post-operative adhesions after digestive surgery: their incidence and prevention: review of the literature. *J. Visc. Surg*. 2012;149(2):e104–14. doi:10.1016/j.jviscsurg.2011.11.006.

[17] Lower, A. M., Hawthorn, R. J., Ellis, H., O'Brien, F., Buchan, S., Crowe, A. M. The impact of adhesions on hospital readmissions over ten years after 8849 open gynaecological operations: an assessment from the Surgical and Clinical Adhesions Research Study. *BJOG*. 2000;107(7):855–62. Available at: http://www.ncbi.nlm.nih.gov/pubmed/10901556. Accessed December 8, 2014.

[18] Hirschelmann, A., Tchartchian, G., Wallwiener, M., Hackethal, A., De Wilde, R. L. A review of the problematic adhesion prophylaxis in gynaecological surgery. *Arch. Gynecol. Obstet*. 2012;285(4):1089–97. doi:10.1007/s00404-011-2097-1.

[19] Cheong, Y. C., Laird, S. M., Shelton, J. B., Ledger, W. L., Li, T. C., Cooke, I. D. The correlation of adhesions and peritoneal fluid cytokine concentrations: a pilot study. *Hum. Reprod*. 2002;17(4):1039–45. Available at: http://www.ncbi.nlm.nih.gov/pubmed/11925402.

[20] Di Saverio, S., Coccolini, F., Galati, M., Smerieri, N., Biffl, W. L., Ansaloni, L., Tugnoli, G., Velmahos, G. C., Sartelli, M., Bendinelli, C., Fraga, G. P., Kelly, M. D., Moore, F. A., Mandalà, V., Mandalà, S., Masetti, M., Jovine, E., Pinna, A. D., Peitzman, A. B., Leppaniemi, A., Sugarbaker, P. H., Goor, H. Van, Moore, E. E., Jeekel, J., Catena, F.

Bologna guidelines for diagnosis and management of adhesive small bowel obstruction (ASBO): 2013 update of the evidence-based guidelines from the world society of emergency surgery ASBO working group. *World J. Emerg. Surg.* 2013;8(1):42. doi:10.1186/1749-7922-8-42.

[21] Radwany, S. M., von Gruenigen, V. E. Palliative and end-of-life care for patients with ovarian cancer. *Clin. Obstet. Gynecol.* 2012;55(1):173–84. doi:10.1097/GRF.0b013e31824b1af1.

[22] Rath, K. S., Loseth, D., Muscarella, P., Phillips, G. S., Fowler, J. M., O'Malley, D. M., Cohn, D. E., Copeland, L. J., Eisenhauer, E. L., Salani, R. Outcomes following percutaneous upper gastrointestinal decompressive tube placement for malignant bowel obstruction in ovarian cancer. *Gynecol. Oncol.* 2013;129(1):103–6. doi:10.1016/j.ygyno.2013.01.021.

[23] Goto, T., Takano, M., Aoyama, T., Miyamoto, M., Watanabe, A., Kato, M., Sasaki, N., Hirata, J., Sasa, H., Furuya, K. Outcomes of palliative bowel surgery for malignant bowel obstruction in patients with gynecological malignancy. *Oncol. Lett.* 2012;4(5):883–888. doi:10.3892/ol.2012.835.

[24] Tunca, J. C., Buchler, D. A., Mack, E. A., Ruzicka, F. F., Crowley, J. J., Carr, W. F. The management of ovarian-cancer-caused bowel obstruction. *Gynecol. Oncol.* 1981;12(2 Pt 1):186–92. Available at: http://www.ncbi.nlm.nih.gov/pubmed/7297929. Accessed November 15, 2013.

[25] Kolomainen, D. F., Daponte, A., Barton, D. P. J., Pennert, K., Ind, T. E. J., Bridges, J. E., Shepherd, J. H., Gore, M. E., Kaye, S. B., Riley, J. Outcomes of surgical management of bowel obstruction in relapsed epithelial ovarian cancer (EOC). *Gynecol. Oncol.* 2012;125(1):31–6. doi:10.1016/j.ygyno.2011.11.007.

[26] Chang, K. H., Brodie, R., Choong, M. A., Sweeney, K. J., Kerin, M. J. Complementary and alternative medicine use in oncology: a questionnaire survey of patients and health care professionals. *BMC Cancer.* 2011;11(1):196. doi:10.1186/1471-2407-11-196.

[27] Gansler, T., Kaw, C., Crammer, C., Smith, T. A population-based study of prevalence of complementary methods use by cancer survivors: a report from the American Cancer Society's studies of cancer survivors. *Cancer.* 2008;113(5):1048–57. doi:10.1002/cncr.23659.

[28] Brauer, J. A., Sehamy, A. El., Metz, J. M., Mao, J. J. Complementary and Alternative Medicine and Supportive Care at Leading Cancer Centers: *J. Altern. Complement. Med.* 2010;16(2):183–186.

[29] Gorman, G., Forest, J., Stapleton, S. J., Hoening, N. A., Marschke, M., Durham, J., Suarez, M. L., Wilkie, D. J. Massage for Cancer Pain: A Study with University and Hospice Collaboration. *J. Hosp. Palliat. Nurs.* 2008;10(4):191–197.

[30] Yates, J. S., Mustian, K. M., Morrow, G. R., Gillies, L. J., Padmanaban, D., Atkins, J. N., Issell, B., Kirshner, J. J., Colman, L. K. Prevalence of complementary and alternative medicine use in cancer patients during treatment. *Support Care Cancer.* 2005;13(10):806–11. doi:10.1007/s 00520-004-0770-7.

[31] Kutner, J. S., Smith, M. C., Corbin, L., Hemphill, L., Benton, K., Mellis, B. K., Beaty, B., Felton, S., Yamashita, T. E., Bryant, L. L., Fairclough, D. L. Massage Therapy versus Simple Touch to Improve Pain and Mood in Patients with Advanced Cancer. *Ann. Intern. Med.* 2008;149(6):369–379.

[32] Williams, A. M., Davies, A., Griffiths, G. Facilitating comfort for hospitalized patients using non-pharmacological measures: preliminary development of clinical practice guidelines. *Int. J. Nurs. Pract.* 2009;15 (3):145–55. doi:10.1111/j.1440-172X.2009.01739.x.

[33] Preece, J. Introducing abdominal massage in palliative care for the relief of constipation. *Complement. Ther. Nurs. Midwifery.* 2002;8(2):101–5. doi:10.1054/ctnm.2002.0610.

[34] Cronfalk, B. S., Strang, P., Ternestedt, B.-M. Inner power, physical strength and existential well-being in daily life: relatives' experiences of receiving soft tissue massage in palliative home care. *J. Clin. Nurs.* 2009;18(15):2225–33. doi:10.1111/j.1365-2702.2008.02517.x.

[35] López-Sendín, N., Alburquerque-Sendín, F., Cleland, J. A., Fernández-de-las-Peñas, C. Effects of physical therapy on pain and mood in patients with terminal cancer: a pilot randomized clinical trial. *J. Altern. Complement. Med.* 2012;18(5):480–6. doi:10.1089/acm.2011.0277.

[36] Di Saverio, S., Coccolini, F., Galati, M., Smerieri, N., Biffl, W. L., Ansaloni, L., Tugnoli, G., Velmahos, G. C., Sartelli, M., Bendinelli, C., Fraga, G. P., Kelly, M. D., Moore, F. A., Mandalà, V., Mandalà, S., Masetti, M., Jovine, E., Pinna, A. D., Peitzman, A. B., Leppaniemi, A., Sugarbaker, P. H., Goor, H. Van, Moore, E. E., Jeekel, J., Catena, F., Van Goor, H. Bologna guidelines for diagnosis and management of adhesive small bowel obstruction (ASBO): 2013 update of the evidence-

based guidelines from the world society of emergency surgery ASBO working group. *World J. Emerg. Surg*. 2013;8(1):42. doi:10.1186/1749-7922-8-42.

[37] Arung, W., Meurisse, M., Detry, O. Pathophysiology and prevention of postoperative peritoneal adhesions. *World J. Gastroenterol*. 2011;17 (41):4545–53. doi:10.3748/wjg.v17.i41.4545.

[38] Yigitler, C., Karakas, I. D. O., Kucukodacı, I. I. Z., Cosar, III A., Bu, I. V. Adhesion-preventing properties of 4% icodextrin and canola oil: a comparative experimental study. 2012;67(11):1303–1308. doi:10.6061/clinics/2012(11)14.

[39] Cheong, Y. C., Shelton, J. B., Laird, S. M., Richmond, M., Kudesia, G., Li, T. C., Ledger, W. L. IL-1, IL-6 and TNF-alpha concentrations in the peritoneal fluid of women with pelvic adhesions. *Hum. Reprod*. 2002;17 (1):69–75. Available at: http://humrep.oxfordjournals.org/content/17/1/69.long.

[40] Ten Broek, R. P. G., Wilbers, J., van Goor, H. Electrocautery causes more ischemic peritoneal tissue damage than ultrasonic dissection. *Surg. Endosc*. 2011;25(6):1827–34. doi:10.1007/s00464-010-1474-3.

[41] Cahill, R. A., Redmond, H. P. Cytokine orchestration in post-operative peritoneal adhesion formation. *World J. Gastroenterol*. 2008;14(31): 4861–6. Available at: http://www.ncbi.nlm.nih.gov/pmc/articles/PMC2739937/pdf/WJG-14-4861.pdf. Accessed July 29, 2014.

[42] Lauder, C. I. W., Garcea, G., Strickland, A., Maddern, G. J. Abdominal adhesion prevention: still a sticky subject? *Dig. Surg*. 2010;27(5):347–58. doi:10.1159/000314805.

[43] Rice, A. D., Reed, E. D., Patterson, K., Wurn, B. F., Wurn, L. J. Clearing bowel obstruction and decreasing pain in a terminally ill patient via manual physical therapy. *J. Palliat. Med*. 2013;16(3):222–3. doi:10.1089/jpm.2012.0458.

[44] Rice, A. D., Wakefield, L. B., Patterson, K., Reed, E. D., Wurn, B. F., King, C. R., Wurn, L. J. Decreasing Adhesions and Avoiding Further Surgery in a Pediatric Patient Involved in a Severe Pedestrian versus Motor Vehicle Accident. *Pediatr. Rep*. 2014;6:5126. Available at: http://www.ncbi.nlm.nih.gov/pmc/articles/PMC3977160/.

[45] Wurn, L. J., Wurn, B. F., King, C. R., Roscow, A. S., Scharf, E. S., Shuster, J. J. Increasing orgasm and decreasing dyspareunia by a manual physical therapy technique. *MedGenMed*. 2004;6(4):47. Available at: http://www.ncbi.nlm.nih.gov/pmc/articles/PMC1480593/. Accessed September 4, 2012.

[46] Rice, A. D., Patterson, K., Wurn, B. F., King, C. R., Wurn, L. J. Update on "Decreasing dyspareunia and dysmenorrhea in women with endometriosis via a manual physical therapy: results from 2 independent studies." *J. Endometr.* 2014;6(3):161–162. doi:10.5301/je.5000193.

[47] Wurn, B. F., Wurn, L. J., Patterson, K., King, C. R., Scharf, E. S. Decreasing dyspareunia and dysmenorrhea in women with endometriosis via a manual physical therapy: Results from two independent studies. *J. Endometr.* 2011;3(4):188–196. doi:10.5301/JE.2012.9088.

[48] Wurn, B. F., Wurn, L. J., King, C. R., Heuer, M. A., Roscow, A. S., Hornberger, K., Scharf, E. S. Treating fallopian tube occlusion with a manual pelvic physical therapy. *Altern. Ther. Heal Med.* 2008;14(1):18–23. Available at: http://www.ncbi.nlm.nih.gov/pubmed/18251317.

[49] Rice, A., King, R., Reed, E., Patterson, K., Wurn, B., Wurn, L. Manual Physical Therapy for Non-Surgical Treatment of Adhesion-Related Small Bowel Obstructions: Two Case Reports. *J. Clin. Med.* 2013;2(1): 1–12. doi:10.3390/jcm2010001.

[50] Wurn, B. F., Wurn, L. J., King, C. R., Heuer, M. A., Roscow, A. S., Scharf, E. S., Shuster, J. J. Treating female infertility and improving IVF pregnancy rates with a manual physical therapy technique. *MedGenMed.* 2004;6(2):51. Available at: http://www.ncbi.nlm.nih.gov/pmc/articles/PMC1395760/. Accessed September 4, 2012.

[51] Wurn, L. J., Wurn, B. F., King, C. R., Roscow, A. S., Scharf, E. S., Shuster, J. J. O-68. *Fertil. Steril.* 2006;86(3):S29–S30. doi:10.1016/j.fertnstert.2006.07.081.

[52] Rice, A. D., Wakefield, L. B., Patterson, K., Reed, E. D., Wurn, B. F., Klingenberg, B., King, C. R., Wurn, L. J. Development and validation of a questionnaire to measure serious and common quality of life issues for patients experiencing small bowel obstructions. *Healthcare.* 2014; 2 (1):139–149. doi:10.3390/healthcare2010139.

[53] Desai, M. J., Kim, A., Fall, P. C., Wang, D. Optimizing Quality of Life Through Palliative Care. *J. Am. Osteopat. Assoc.* 2007;107(12):ES9–ES14.

Index

A

abdominal surgery, vii, xi, 111, 113, 118
access, x, 51, 59, 63, 88, 98, 108, 112
accounting, 12
achlorhydria, 103
acidosis, 3
AD, 96, 121, 122, 124
additives, 114
adenocarcinoma, 20, 110
adhesiolysis, x, 88, 98, 127
adhesion(s), vii, ix, x, xi, 87, 98, 101, 102, 107, 113, 114, 115, 116, 117, 118, 119, 120, 121, 123, 125, 126, 127, 128, 129, 130, 132, 134, 136, 139
adhesive capsulitis, 116
adults, 5, 7, 30, 88, 93, 95, 96, 116
advancement, 12, 21, 90
adverse effects, 33
adverse event, 64, 132, 134
aesthetic, 94
aetiology, viii, 10, 11, 12, 16, 17, 19, 24, 25
afferent loop obstruction, vii, x, 97, 102, 108, 110, 111, 112
Africa, 6
age, ix, 6, 12, 13, 16, 17, 18, 20, 22, 32, 41, 42, 43, 53, 57, 60, 65, 66, 71, 128, 132
ageing population, 13
algorithm, 26, 92
alternative medicine, 127, 137, 138
amputation, 2
analgesic, 47
anastomosis, 24, 79, 102, 107, 108, 112
anatomy, 11, 13, 25, 27, 90
anchoring, 16, 17
anemia, 5, 103, 104
angiogenesis, 126, 135
anorexia, 5
antibiotic, 60
antispasmodics, 47
anus, 3, 20
aorta, x, 98, 105
apathy, 38
apex, 14, 41, 42, 43, 44, 45
appendectomy, 62
appendicitis, 62
Aristotle, 97, 112
artery, x, 98, 105
ascending colon, 62
ascites, 78, 83, 84, 85, 106
aspiration, 91
assessment, viii, 20, 29, 31, 33, 35, 41, 43, 44, 45, 108, 134, 136
asymptomatic, 12, 19, 23, 26, 28
attachment, 14
avoidance, 118
awareness, 10, 18

B

back pain, 117
bacteremia, 74
barium, 4, 21, 49, 50, 51, 52, 56, 61, 67, 68, 69, 70, 71, 74, 79, 89, 90, 104, 108
barium enema, 4, 49, 51, 56, 61, 67, 68, 69, 71, 79, 89, 90
barriers, xi, 10, 114, 127
benefits, xi, 23, 25, 114, 115, 117, 118
benign, x, 20, 98, 99, 101, 107
bezoars, x, 98, 101
BI, 111
bile, 99, 103, 107
bile acids, 103
bile duct, 107
biliary atresia, 110
Bilious vomiting, vii, 1, 2
Billroth II, x, 97, 99, 100, 102, 107, 108
biofeedback, 23, 29
biopsy, 106
bleeding, 2, 3, 4, 18, 19, 20, 36
blood, 4, 6, 16, 19, 36, 37, 38, 41, 42, 43, 44, 59, 66, 82
blood flow, 19, 41, 42, 43, 44, 66
blood supply, 82
blood vessels, 16
bones, 13
bowel perforation, 42, 56, 94, 105, 115

C

calcifications, 78
caliber, 106
cancer, vii, x, xi, xii, 98, 102, 103, 111, 125, 126, 127, 128, 129, 131, 132, 133, 134, 135, 137, 138
cancer stem cells, 135
candidates, xii, 43, 45, 61, 123, 125, 127
capillary, 6
carbon, 91
carbon dioxide, 91
carcinoma, 126
case study, 122
cecum, 38, 61, 92
cervical cancer, 135
cervical radiculopathy, 122
challenges, 10
chemical, 89
chemotherapy, xi, 2, 125, 126, 128, 132
Chicago, 7
childhood, 28, 67, 68, 69, 73, 95
children, vii, viii, 1, 2, 3, 4, 5, 6, 7, 12, 18, 20, 31, 32, 33, 34, 35, 37, 39, 41, 44, 48, 57, 60, 61, 63, 64, 65, 66, 67, 68, 69, 70, 71, 72, 73, 74, 77, 95, 119
chloral, 46
cholangitis, 103
classification, ix, 77, 79, 132
clinical diagnosis, 21
clinical presentation, 38
clinical symptoms, 38, 43, 115
clinical syndrome, viii, 9
clinical trials, 118
coccyx, 13, 14
collaboration, 10
collagen, 12, 16, 114
colon, 20, 28, 38, 47, 79, 90
colon cancer, 20, 28
color, 43, 66
colorectal surgeon, 10, 11
common symptoms, 2
compilation, x, 88
complex interactions, 11
complexity, 11, 16
compliance, 17
complications, 25, 28, 30, 43, 45, 46, 62, 94, 111, 127, 136
compression, x, 98, 101, 131
computed tomography, 37, 90
connective tissue, 18
consensus, 26, 32, 35, 93
constipation, viii, 9, 11, 18, 20, 22, 23, 24, 127, 138
construction, x, 97, 99, 109
contracture, 122
controlled studies, 47
controlled trials, 21
controversial, 133

controversies, 70
cooperation, 11
correlation, 43, 55, 65, 73, 136
cost, 33, 94
covering, 15
cranium, 116
CRP, 38, 41, 42, 43
CT, x, 2, 39, 40, 43, 44, 61, 65, 90, 98, 104, 105, 111
CT scan, 90, 106
culture, 59
CV, 83
cystic fibrosis, 12
cytokines, 64

D

data collection, 64
database, 63
deaths, 36, 126
defecation, viii, 9, 17, 18, 23, 25, 28, 29, 30
defects, 17, 101, 106
deficiency, 22, 27, 103, 104
deficit, 22
deformation, 116, 119, 128
dehydration, 42, 45, 46, 131
dementia, 18
detectable, 36
detection, 35, 36, 61, 66, 71, 84
developed countries, 3
developing countries, 2
diagnostic criteria, viii, 23, 29, 31, 35, 36
diaphragm, 14, 15
diarrhea, 3, 4, 5, 104
diet, 92, 115, 118, 129, 131, 133
differential diagnosis, 3, 105
dilation, 78, 106, 107, 109, 117
discomfort, 13, 19, 104
disease progression, 127, 134
diseases, 12, 59, 111
disorder, viii, 10, 11, 19, 20, 22, 25, 70, 78
distribution, 132, 133
doctors, 34
draft, 34
drainage, 106, 107
drugs, 59
duodenum, 99
dysmenorrhea, 123, 140
dyspareunia, 123, 139, 140
dyspnea, 4

E

edema, 58, 60, 92, 131, 134
editors, 83
Egypt, 94
Ehlers-Danlos syndrome, 18
elderly population, 25
electricity, 88
electromyography, 22
e-mail, 125
emergency, x, 34, 39, 40, 59, 73, 98, 102, 104, 110, 119, 122, 137, 139
Emergency Room, ix, 87
endometriosis, 123, 140
endoscopic retrograde cholangiopancreatography, 112
endoscopy, 109
enema(s), viii, ix, 3, 4, 31, 32, 35, 36, 38, 39, 40, 42, 43, 44, 45, 46, 47, 48, 49, 51, 52, 53, 54, 55, 56, 57, 58, 59, 60, 61, 67, 68, 69, 70, 71, 72, 73, 74, 79, 88, 89, 90, 92, 93, 94, 95
energy, 128
England, 70
enteritis, x, 98, 101, 102, 103, 106, 109, 118
enterocoele, 25
enteroliths, x, 98
entrapment, x, 98, 101
environment(s), 33, 48, 63
epidemiology, 13, 33, 120
epigastrium, 3
epithelial ovarian cancer, 137
epithelium, 15
equipment, 43
ethics, 124
ethnic groups, 13
ethnicity, 13
etiology, vii, x, xi, 83, 88, 113, 125
Europe, 50, 51

evacuation, 17, 19, 23, 26
evidence, viii, 21, 22, 31, 32, 33, 43, 44, 47, 57, 58, 61, 62, 65, 119, 122, 137, 138
evolution, 30, 65, 74
examinations, 6
excision, x, 24, 98, 107, 108, 109, 126
excretion, 106
expenditures, 115
expertise, 40, 48
exposure, 39, 40, 44, 48, 68, 114

F

faecal incontinence, viii, 9, 11, 18, 22, 24
families, 63
family history, 20
fascia, 14, 16, 17
fear, 104
feces, 38, 49
femur, 2
fever, 6, 37
fixation, 25, 62
fluid, x, 41, 43, 44, 45, 46, 66, 98, 105, 121, 136, 139
Foley catheter, 92
food, 104
force, 17, 91, 92, 94, 116, 126, 128
formation, xi, 91, 113, 114, 115, 116, 118, 119, 120, 121, 125, 126, 127, 128, 134, 136, 139

G

gangrene, ix, 77, 103
gastrectomy, x, 97, 99, 100, 102, 105, 106, 110, 111
gastric outlet obstruction, 111
gastritis, 2
gastroenteritis, 2
gastroenterostomy, 111
gastrointestinal surgical procedures, x, 88
gastrojejunostomy, x, 97, 99, 101, 107, 110, 112
general anesthesia, 46, 67
general surgeon, x, 34, 88
gestation, 79
glucagon, 47, 67, 68
grades, 26
grading, 21, 29
grants, 90
Greece, 1, 97, 112
growth, 119, 126
guidance, viii, 32, 45, 49, 67, 68, 69, 74, 120
guidelines, vii, viii, ix, 11, 31, 32, 33, 34, 35, 36, 41, 50, 56, 63, 64, 66, 115, 121, 122, 137, 138

H

hair, 15
hair follicle, 15
healing, xi, 113, 114, 118, 126
health, xi, 10, 23, 47, 51, 62, 63, 113, 115, 116, 137
health care, xi, 10, 113, 137
health care professionals, 10, 137
health insurance, 47, 51, 62, 63
heavy metals, 88
hematoma, 39
Henoch-Schonlein purpura, 61
hernia, 16, 102, 106, 109, 110
herniation, x, 98, 101, 102
histological examination, 19
history, viii, ix, xi, 2, 4, 6, 10, 11, 13, 18, 20, 21, 22, 43, 87, 88, 101, 114, 118, 127, 129, 130, 131, 134
hospitalization, 62
human, 33
humanism, 124
hydrops, 84
hypersensitivity, 19
hypothesis, 19
hypovolemia, 3, 45
hypovolemic shock, 61
hysterectomy, 126

I

identification, 28, 62, 116
idiopathic, 29, 45, 92, 93
ileum, 62, 78, 117
image(s), 21, 27, 37, 49, 105
imaging modalities, 12
immunization, 64
improvements, xi, 10, 114, 119, 134
in utero, 78
incidence, 6, 12, 13, 16, 17, 35, 37, 38, 42, 43, 44, 61, 78, 91, 102, 103, 106, 120, 136
independence, xi, 114
India, 85
individuals, 11, 12
induction, 119
infancy, 11, 67, 68, 70, 72
infants, vii, ix, 1, 2, 3, 6, 7, 32, 35, 37, 38, 42, 52, 53, 57, 58, 63, 64, 67, 70, 71, 72, 95
infection, 114, 131
infertility, 115, 116, 123, 140
inflammation, xi, 113, 114, 126, 135
inflammatory bowel disease, 19
ingest, 21
ingestion, 4, 88
initiation, 20, 36, 131
injury, 62, 114
insertion, x, 14, 98, 107, 110, 112
institutions, 39, 52, 59, 92, 93
integrity, 10, 15, 17, 22
interference, 82
intervention, x, xi, 21, 74, 88, 95, 107, 114, 115, 126, 135
intestinal atresia, ix, 77, 78, 79, 82, 83, 84, 85
intestinal obstruction, 49, 78, 79, 82, 134, 135
intestine, ix, 78, 83, 87, 99
intravenous fluids, xi, 113
intravenously, 45
intussuception, vii, 16
intussuscipiens, vii, 1, 84, 88
invagination, vii, 1, 43, 44, 84, 85, 90
iodinated contrast, 49
ionising radiation, 21
iron, 103, 104
irritability, 36, 37, 38, 117
irritable bowel syndrome, 18
ischemia, 2, 4, 41, 42, 43, 61, 66, 78
isolation, 10, 43
issues, 124, 140

J

Japan, ix, 31, 32, 34, 35, 39, 40, 46, 47, 48, 49, 50, 51, 52, 53, 56, 58, 59, 60, 62, 63, 64, 83
jaundice, 112
jejunum, 78, 99

L

laminar, 14
laparoscopic surgery, 74, 102
laparoscopy, x, 74, 88, 93, 94, 95
laparotomy, x, 61, 88, 93, 94, 95, 120
large intestine, 104
latency, 22, 29
lead, ix, 6, 17, 39, 41, 69, 73, 78, 82, 84, 87, 92, 93, 94, 95, 103
lesions, 18, 106
lethargy, vii, 1, 6, 38, 64
levator, 14, 16, 17, 27
life cycle, 29
ligament, 15
lipid peroxides, 64
liquids, 129
liver, 110
liver transplant, 110
liver transplantation, 110
longevity, 118
low risk, 119
lumen, viii, x, 9, 89, 93, 98, 105
lying, 99
lymph, 71, 101, 106
lymph node, 71, 101
lymphadenopathy, 106

lymphoma, 2, 74
lysis, 114

M

magnetic resonance, 17, 37
magnetic resonance imaging, 17, 37
majority, 51, 53, 54, 63, 78, 79
malignancy, xi, xii, 19, 88, 93, 104, 125, 126, 137
malnutrition, 103, 115
manipulation, xi, 114, 116, 128
manual movement, 128
mass, vii, x, xi, 1, 2, 3, 4, 5, 37, 38, 89, 92, 93, 98, 104, 105, 125, 126, 130, 131
MDCT, x, 98, 105
measurement(s), 21, 22, 28, 118, 119
meconium, 78, 79, 84, 85
media, viii, 31, 35, 42, 45, 47, 49, 50, 51, 52, 55, 56, 60, 70
median, 5, 12, 16, 60, 102, 107
medical, vii, ix, xii, 2, 4, 5, 6, 18, 33, 35, 48, 59, 63, 87, 88, 93, 126, 129, 130
medical history, 6, 129, 130
medication, 68, 118, 131
medicine, 33, 77, 124, 136
meningitis, vii, 1
mesenteric vessels, 106
mesentery, 79, 89, 92
meta-analysis, 52, 73
metabolic acidosis, 38
metastasis, 2
methodology, 23, 93
models, 88, 116
modifications, 36, 116, 127, 128
moisture, 128
Montenegro, 122
morbidity, 3, 7, 24, 49, 88, 108, 127
morphine, 46
morphometric, 16
mortality, 3, 7, 20, 88, 108, 127
mortality rate, 127
MR, 29, 85
MRI, 21, 22, 29
mucosa, 15, 19
mucus, 4, 18, 19
multivariate analysis, 134
muscle relaxant, 47
muscles, 14, 15, 17, 23, 25, 28

N

nasogastric tube, 91, 126
necrosis, viii, 31, 32, 38, 41, 42, 43, 44, 62, 89, 92
neonates, 79
nerve, 15, 16, 22, 25, 29
neurological disease, 12
neuropathy, 22
nodes, 102
non-malignant bowel obstruction, vii, xii, 126
non-surgical therapy, 94
North America, 50, 51
nutrition, 129, 131, 134

O

obstruction, vii, ix, x, xi, xii, 1, 41, 66, 83, 87, 93, 97, 99, 101, 103, 104, 105, 106, 107, 108, 110, 111, 112, 114, 115, 117, 121, 125, 126, 127, 129, 131, 133, 135
occlusion, ix, 77, 79, 82, 112, 123, 140
occult blood, 4, 7, 36, 38, 64
ODS, 29
oedema, 19
oil, 121, 139
omentum, 49
opacification, 79
opacity, 38
operations, x, 24, 25, 97, 99, 102, 136
orchestration, 121, 139
organ(s), 13, 21, 27, 30, 114, 128
orgasm, 123, 139
osteopathic manual therapy, xi, 114
outpatient, 59
ovarian cancer, 127, 134, 135, 137
oxygen, 50, 52, 70

P

paediatric patients, 18
pain, vii, x, xii, 1, 2, 3, 4, 5, 6, 19, 36, 37, 38, 88, 92, 104, 115, 116, 117, 118, 122, 126, 127, 128, 129, 130, 131, 132, 133, 138, 139
palliative, xi, 107, 125, 127, 128, 129, 130, 132, 133, 134, 135, 137, 138
pancreas, 106, 131
pancreatic cancer, 103, 107, 111
pancreaticoduodenectomy, x, 97, 99, 101, 103, 105, 106, 107, 109, 111, 112
pancreatitis, 103, 104, 110, 111, 112
paradigm shift, x, 88
parasitic infection, 12
parents, 2
pathogenesis, 61
pathology, 11, 12, 18, 19, 20, 21, 91, 94, 106
pathophysiological, viii, 10
pathophysiology, vii, viii, x, 3, 9, 11, 15, 17, 25, 28, 41, 88
pediatrician, vii, 1
pelvic floor, viii, 9, 10, 11, 12, 13, 14, 15, 16, 17, 18, 19, 20, 21, 23, 25, 27, 29
pelvic surgery, xi, 113, 115, 120, 130
pelvis, xi, 13, 114, 116, 118, 125, 126, 129, 132
percentile, 5
perforation, viii, ix, 31, 32, 42, 49, 52, 53, 56, 57, 61, 62, 69, 72, 83, 84, 87, 89, 91, 103, 104
perineum, 13, 17, 24
peristalsis, 88, 92, 93
peritoneal cavity, 52, 78, 83
peritoneum, 13, 15, 49, 93, 101
peritonitis, 4, 42, 43, 44, 49, 58, 61, 62, 69, 70, 82, 84, 85, 89, 91, 103, 104, 115, 127
Philadelphia, 83
physical activity, 23
physical therapy, vii, xi, xii, 114, 116, 119, 122, 123, 126, 127, 128, 129, 133, 134, 138, 139, 140
physicians, 4, 49, 115, 134
physiology, 11, 22, 25, 27
pilot study, 136
plexus, 16
PLP, 39, 43, 44, 60, 61
population, 12, 19, 20, 45, 66, 78, 88, 89, 93, 94, 118, 119, 132, 134, 135, 137
post-surgical adhesions, xi, 114
precedent, 119
predictability, 114
pregnancy, 79, 83, 85, 123, 140
preservation, 82
pressure gauge, 52
preterm infants, 83
prevention, 114, 120, 121, 133, 136, 139
primary tumor, 2
procidentia, 11, 17
prognosis, 79, 126
prolapse, 3, 11, 12, 13, 16, 17, 18, 19, 20, 24, 25, 26, 27, 28, 30
prolapsed, 3, 20, 21, 30, 88
prophylaxis, 136
pseudocyst, 78, 85
psychiatric illness, 12
psychological problems, 10, 19, 26
pubis, 14
P-value, 133

Q

quality of life, viii, xi, xii, 9, 10, 24, 114, 115, 118, 119, 124, 126, 127, 131, 140
questionnaire, ix, 32, 34, 118, 124, 131, 137, 140

R

radiation, x, xi, 22, 39, 40, 44, 48, 90, 98, 101, 102, 103, 106, 109, 110, 112, 118, 125, 126, 128, 129, 130, 132
radiation treatment, 128, 130, 132
radiculopathy, 116
radiography, 57, 64, 79
RE, 112
reactions, 131

reading, viii, 9
recognition, 6
recommendations, 32, 33, 127, 134
reconstruction, x, 28, 97, 99, 100, 101, 102, 107, 108, 109, 110, 111, 112
rectal prolapse, viii, 3, 9, 11, 12, 13, 16, 17, 18, 19, 20, 22, 25, 26, 27, 28, 29, 30
rectal wall, viii, 3, 9, 15, 16, 17, 25
rectocele, 27
rectosigmoid, 3, 15, 42
rectum, ix, 3, 4, 11, 14, 15, 16, 17, 18, 19, 20, 21, 24, 25, 27, 32, 52
recurrence, x, 5, 24, 25, 59, 60, 61, 62, 70, 74, 98, 101, 103, 106
relatives, 138
relief, 104, 138
remission, xii, 126
repair, 26, 107, 108, 109, 114
requirements, 24, 131
resection, 24, 30, 42, 43, 49, 61, 62, 79, 88, 89, 92, 93, 94, 112, 115, 127
resolution, 39, 60, 115, 116, 117, 118, 119
resources, 13, 24, 115
response, ix, xi, 24, 32, 34, 87, 113, 114, 125, 131
restrictions, 129, 133
risk(s), ix, xi, 5, 12, 13, 24, 25, 32, 42, 43, 49, 53, 57, 61, 66, 74, 114, 115, 116, 120, 127
risk factors, 12, 13, 57, 120
Roux-en-Y reconstruction, x, 97, 99, 100, 101, 102, 107, 108, 109, 110, 111, 112

S

safety, x, 45, 72, 88
salmon, 4
SBO, vii, xi, 1, 113, 114, 115, 116, 117, 118, 119, 127, 129, 131, 132, 133, 134
scar tissue, 114, 119
school, 129
scope, 91
secretin, 106, 107, 111
seeding, 93
sensation, 17, 19
sensitivity, 37, 39, 40, 43
sensory modalities, 23
sepsis, ix, 25, 41, 59, 61, 87, 91
septic shock, 38, 42
septum, 16, 25
services, 24
sexual activity, 13
shape, 15, 16
shear, 128
shock, viii, 6, 31, 32, 41, 44, 62
showing, 89, 90, 107, 117
side effects, 24, 116, 117, 127
sigmoid colon, 3, 15, 16, 20
signs, 3, 4, 6, 36, 38, 42, 60, 65, 67, 92
Sinai, 87
sinuses, 15
skin, 13, 15
small bowel obstruction, vii, ix, xi, 39, 44, 57, 87, 88, 93, 114, 120, 121, 122, 124, 127, 128, 137, 138, 140
smooth muscle, 16
smooth muscle cells, 16
society, 35, 122, 137, 139
solid tumors, 126
solubility, 103
solution, 52, 68, 127
specialists, 10
species, 29
sphincter, 22
spine, 14
splinting, 123
SS, 28, 29
stasis, 104
state, 2, 41, 42, 43
statistics, 35, 122
steatorrhea, 103, 104
stenosis, x, 83, 84, 98, 106, 107, 108, 112
stent, x, 98, 107, 109, 110, 112, 127
sterile, 78, 83, 92
stomach, 109
stretching, 17, 22, 106
strictures, 111
structure, 14, 17, 82
success rate, ix, 32, 35, 42, 43, 45, 50, 51, 55, 57, 58

sulfate, 47, 70
Sun, 26
surface area, 14
surgical intervention, ix, xi, 23, 87, 90, 113, 116, 119, 127, 132
surgical technique, x, xi, 88, 114, 127
survival, 70, 107, 127, 131
survivors, 103, 137
suture, 25
sweat, 15
symptomology, 127
symptoms, vii, viii, xii, 1, 3, 4, 5, 9, 10, 11, 12, 18, 19, 20, 21, 23, 26, 29, 36, 37, 38, 39, 41, 42, 43, 57, 60, 67, 94, 104, 115, 116, 118, 119, 126, 129, 131, 133, 134
syndrome, viii, 9, 16, 17, 18, 19, 22, 25, 27, 28, 29, 61, 110, 111

T

target, 38, 39, 60, 78, 90, 91, 114
techniques, x, 10, 17, 25, 50, 88, 93, 94, 116, 128
temperature, 128
tendon, 17
tension, 52
terminally ill, 139
testicle, 118
testing, 4, 7, 22, 29, 36, 64
texture, 128
therapist, 128
therapy, ix, xi, xii, 6, 24, 29, 59, 87, 95, 114, 115, 117, 123, 126, 127, 128, 132, 134
thoracotomy, 2
thrombosis, 79
tissue, 18, 38, 114, 116, 121, 122, 128, 138, 139
TNF, 121, 139
TNF-alpha, 121, 139
toddlers, vii, 1
training, 39, 48
transverse colon, 3
transverse section, 16
trauma, 93, 114, 118, 120, 136
trial, 23, 70, 138
tumor, 93, 106, 131

U

UK, 9
ulcer, 16, 19, 27, 28
ultrasonography, 22, 65, 66, 85, 90
ultrasound, 3, 6, 37, 61, 68, 69, 72, 78, 79, 84, 89, 122
United, ix, xi, 87, 113
United States, ix, xi, 87, 113
urethra, 14
USA, 113, 123
uterine cancer, 126

V

vagina, 14, 18, 21
validation, 118, 124, 131, 133, 140
variations, 16, 27
vector, 17
vessels, 15
viral gastroenteritis, 88
viscera, 14, 17, 116, 128
visualization, 91
volvulus, x, 78, 83, 98, 101
vomiting, vii, ix, 1, 2, 3, 5, 6, 36, 37, 38, 77, 79, 91, 104

W

Wales, 70, 75
water, viii, 31, 32, 35, 49, 51, 52, 69, 89, 95
weakness, 12, 17
weight loss, 20, 104
well-being, 138
wheezing, 4
white blood cell count, 42, 43
workload, 121